PHARM.D. TO M.D.

FROM PHARMACY SCHOOL TO MEDICAL SCHOOL

A COMPLETE GUIDE TO GETTING INTO MEDICAL SCHOOL

Nathan M. Gartland, PharmD

PHARM.D. TO M.D.

Copyright © 2021 Nathan M. Gartland

All rights reserved. This book is protected under the copyright laws of the United States of America. Any reproduction or other unauthorized use of the material is herein prohibited.

Disclaimer: This publication is designed to provide accurate and authoritative information with regard to the subject matter covered. The information in this book is not intended to replace or conflict with the financial or academic advice provided by your designated professional(s) and may not be suitable for your personal situation. The ultimate decision to make any changes regarding your finances or medical school application should be determined only by you and or your designated advisor. The contents of this book are the views and opinions of the author only. The author disclaims all liability in connection with the use of this book. I am not a financial advisor or academic counselor.

The author does not own the rights to any external resource referenced throughout this book and is not responsible for the quality of information, put forth by external sources. The author also receives no financial compensation from any of the recommended external sources or third-party content and is strictly an advocate from personal experience. I absolve myself from any liability including advice associated with outside references.

Editor: Jacob Nannen

PHARM.D. TO M.D.

DEDICATION

To my parents whose love and faith in me have made all of this possible. Thank you for being my inspiration. To my best friend and girlfriend Julia for her constant encouragement to chase my dreams.

"Don't be afraid to start over again. This time you're not starting from scratch, you're starting from experience."

PHARM.D. TO M.D.

WHY YOU SHOULD READ THIS BOOK:

Before we dissect this complex process, allow me to introduce myself. My name is Nathan Gartland and I am a second year medical student, also known as an MS2, and a licensed pharmacist. Prior to my acceptance to an allopathic medical program, I was a pharmacy student at Duquesne University, in Pittsburgh Pennsylvania.

The thought of going to medical school had always been looming in the back of my mind but doing so seemed like an unreachable goal. I had already committed myself to a professional career in pharmacy and making the switch seemed impossible. I kept asking myself, "What would my classmates think? What would my parents think? Is this a terrible idea? Where do I even start?" Following the age-old saying, "If it ain't broke, don't try to fix it," I thought, "why should I abandon a career in pharmacy when it is going so well for me?" You may be asking yourself these very same questions.

As I progressed through my schooling, I became restless with the reality that I would end up having to complete a pharmacy residency to work with patients. While this isn't entirely true anymore – considering the growth of the profession – the dept of patient care management would still fall short. It wasn't until my second professional year of school that the possibility of pursuing a career in both pharmacy and medicine dawned upon me. This dream didn't come to fruition until I received insight from my personal mentor, Dr. Brandon Smith, PharmD, MD, and a fellow pharmacy student, Dr. Tess Calcagno PharmD, who both underwent this very same transition.

If you are reading this paragraph right now, you have already taken the first steps on this incredible journey. When I began this difficult transition, I found myself at the mercy of the application cycle. I had no in-house guidance, received no academic counseling, and pushed through the cycle by the "seat of my pants." While there is a plethora of online resources available to applicants, there are very few references that provide a comprehensive look at how to get into medical school. If they do, it will likely cost you thousands of dollars to get past the paywall. Additionally, none of these resources provide important instructions or perspectives that would benefit pharmacy students. Then again, why would they? Most authors have never been to pharmacy school and neither have most medical school applicants. I wrote this book to provide you, the 1% of medical school applicants, with the necessary input to conquer the application cycle and to successfully receive a medical school acceptance. My only goal is to make your application cycle far easier to get through than mine was.

While much of the information provided in this book is far from novel, I hope it will be a useful resource to guide you through this isolating process. You will find yourself torn in many different directions as your pharmacy school responsibilities clash with your application tasks. Stay focused on your final goals and you can accomplish anything. You are already qualified enough to make it into pharmacy school and survive the academic rigors. Therefore, you are more than equipped to get into the medical school of your dreams.

We will address the different components of the application cycle in the chronological order that will best suit your cycle needs. You may find yourself further along in the process than other readers so feel free to jump around to a section of your choosing.

We will cover various pitfalls along the way to make sure you avoid costly mistakes that will hurt your checkbook and chances of getting an acceptance. We will cover pharmacy specific factors unbeknownst to traditional applicants including APPE rotation recommendations, pharmacy licensure boards (NAPLEX and MPJE), and more! Join me on this tremendous undertaking and follow along as we take your dream from inception to reality.

NATHAN M. GARTLAND

Welcome to my personal medical school application crash course, constructed from a pharmacist's perspective.

PHARM.D. TO M.D.

TABLE OF CONTENTS:

WHY YOU SHOULD READ THIS BOOK: 7

PART ONE: THE MEDICAL SCHOOL BLUEPRINT   15
  1. WOULD YOU EVEN MAKE THE CUT?   18
  2. APPLYING TO MEDICAL SCHOOL IS EXPENSIVE: 22
  3. CHOOSING A MEDICAL SCPECIALTY: 30
  4. MAKE AN AAMC ACCOUNT: 35
  5. REACH OUT TO YOUR UNIVERSITY'S PRE-HEALH ADVISORS: 36
  6. TAKE THE MCAT FIRST AND TAKE IT SERIOUSLY: 37
  7. YOUR PHARM.D. IS YOUR MOST PRIZED POCESSION: 39

PART TWO: THE SCHEDULE   41
  UNDERGRADUATE YEARS: 43
  PROFESSIONAL YEAR ONE (PY1):   44
  PROFESSIONAL YEAR TWO (PY2):   46
  PROFESSIONAL YEAR THREE (PY3):   50
  PROFESSIONAL YEAR FOUR (PY4):   58

PART THREE: THE MCAT   63
  THE PHARMACY STUDENT STRUGGLE: 64
  MY MCAT BACKGROUND: 66
  GETTING TO KNOW THE MCAT: 67
  HOW THE MCAT IS SCORED: 68
  GETTING STARTED: 69
  DEVELOP A PLAN: 79
  VOIDING YOUR MCAT: 84

PART FOUR: THE PRIMARY APPLICATION — 87

- PRIMARY APPLICATION TIMELINE AND THE PERKS OF APPLYING EARLY: — 88
- BUILDING A STRONG APPLICATION: — 92
- THE PRIMARY APPLICATION LAYOUT: — 98

PART FIVE: SECONDARY APPLICATIONS — 141

- SECONDARY OVERVIEW: — 142
- PRE-WRITE YOUR SECONDARY APPLICATIONS: — 143
- COMMON SECONDARY PROMPTS: — 145
- SECONDARY ESSAY TIMING: — 149

PART SIX: THE CASPER EXAM — 151

- ALTUS SUITE COMPONENTS: — 152
- AAMC SITUATIONAL JUDGMENT TEST (SJT): — 163

PART SEVEN: OSTEOPATHIC SCHOOLS OF MEDICINE — 165

- OSTEOPATHIC PHYSICIAN OVERVIEW: — 166
- OSTEOPATHIC MEDICINE LIMITATIONS: — 166
- SHOULD YOU APPLY TO D.O. SCHOOLS: — 170
- MAKING YOUR D.O. SCHOOL LIST: — 173
- AACOMAS: OSTEOPATHIC MEDICINE APPLICATION SERVICE: — 175

PART EIGHT: THE INTERVIEW — 179

- THE INTERVIEW TIMELINE — 181
- THE PHARMACY ADVANTAGE: — 182
- DIFFERENT INTERVIEW TYPES & STRATEGIES: — 182
- INTERVIEW PREPARATION: — 187
- QUESTIONS TO EXPECT: — 190
- THANK YOU LETTERS: — 194

PART NINE: THE PRE/POST-INTERVIEW LIMBO — 199
UNDERSTANDING WAITLISTS: — 200
PROVIDE UPDATE LETTERS TO PROGRAMS: — 202
LETTER OF INTENT (LOI): — 207
NO FORMAL UNDERGRADUATE DEGREE: — 209
PHARMACY REDICNECY APPLICATIONS: — 209

PART TEN: HOLDING A MEDICAL SCHOOL ACCEPTANCE — 213
ACCEPTING YOUR ACCEPTANCE: — 214
PHARMACY BOARDS: — 215
PHARMACY SCHOOL V.S. MEDICAL SCHOOL: — 216
PREPARING FOR THE WORST: — 218

ADDITIONAL RESOURCES: — 219
MD-PHD PROGRAM: — 219
TEXAS MEDICAL & DENTAL SCHOOLS APPLICATION SERVICE (TMDSAS): — 220
CARIBBEAN MEDICAL SCHOOLS: — 221
MUST READ SUPPLEMENTAL CONTENT: — 223

CLOSING REMARKS: — 225
ABOUT THE AUTHOR: — 227
CHAPTER REFERENCES: — 229

PHARM.D. TO M.D.

PART ONE:

THE MEDICAL SCHOOL BLUEPRINT

"The aim of medicine is to prevent disease and prolong life; the ideal of medicine is to eliminate the need of a physician."

– William J. Mayo

Every year the number of medical school applicants has gradually risen yet the number of available medical student seats has remained relatively fixed. This statistic may not seem like that big of a deal to many of this book's readers, but it should highlight the reality that getting into medical school is getting harder and harder each year. One may ask, "How can this be?" It is certainly a multifactorial phenomenon, but the following are likely the largest contributors. The steady growth in the utilization of test prep resources, a surge in more qualified "gap-year" applicants, and tactical application planning. The latter of which I will be focusing on during this chapter.

If you are reading this book, you are likely already a strong and motivated pharmacy student interested in pursuing a career in medicine. You may ask; "Why would I need to follow the same rulebook as a traditional pre-health applicant? Isn't my unique educational background sufficient to set me apart from the rest of the crowd?" Perhaps it is, but in my experience, it certainly is not. Applying to medical school has many moving parts that require varying degrees of attention. Your educational background will pique an admission board's interest, but it won't occupy them for long if you have neglected other important parts of the application. We will discuss all of these in the coming chapters, but your first goal should be to understand the big picture. Know that your pharmacy education can be a fantastic asset to your application, but it will not allow you to coast through the cycle. Please do not be deceived into believing that your prior education affords you a free pass to getting into medical school.

You will need to actively learn about the application process and collect as much information as you can. You do not just learn how to drive a car by jumping behind the wheel and hoping the ride goes smoothly. Well, I am sure that some readers may argue that the aforementioned approach may be the best way to learn but I am here to argue that it is certainly not the safest. Normally, you would participate in a driver's education course, learn the laws of the road, and practice driving while supervised before going out on the open road. Applying to medical school has many parallels to this simple analogy. Unfortunately, pharmacy students and other non-traditional applicants lack this crucial supervision component. Traditional pre-medical students tend to have support and guidance from their institution's advisory program, a resource unbeknownst to their pharmacy peers. As a pharmacy student you are often applying with half the information you need (at best) or completely blind (at worst). Driving a car without the gift of vision can be cause for some disastrous results. Learn to walk before you run, learn to plan before you apply. "Success is when opportunity meets preparation."

Before we dive into the intricacies of the medical school application, let me first highlight some of the major principles that will create a strong application foundation. Use these principles as the infrastructure for your application. You may want to refer to this chapter later to remind yourself if you get lost along the way. Benjamin Franklin once famously said, "by failing to prepare, you are preparing to fail." Build your information arsenal, study the approach, have a plan, and stick to it!

KEY PRINCIPLES:

1. **WOULD YOU EVEN MAKE THE CUT:**

2. **APPLYING TO MEDICAL SCHOOL IS EXPENSIVE:**

3. **CHOOSING A MEDICAL SPECIALTY:**

4. **CREATE YOUR AAMC ACCOUNT:**

5. **CONTACT YOUR UNIVERSITY'S PRE-HEALTH OFFICE:**

6. **TAKE THE MCAT FIRST AND TAKE IT SERIOUSLY:**

7. **YOUR PHARM.D. IS YOUR MOST PRIZED POCESSION:**

1. WOULD YOU EVEN MAKE THE CUT?

You are probably wondering what it takes to even get into medical school. Of course, good grades and a passion for medicine go a long way but what does that really mean? I certainly had no idea when I began to investigate this career altering pathway. What I have found is that heartfelt personal statements, stellar letters of recommendations, and fascinating clinical activities often fall to the wayside when an applicant has low medical school statistics. Let that last sentence sink in. As pharmacy applicants those facets of a good application are our bread and butter. We have ample clinical experience, a laundry list of meaningful patient encounters, and access to devoted professors. I am here to tell you that these are ancillary components, at least in the beginning stages. Your final goal may be to get an acceptance, but your short-term goal is to survive the first round of application rejections. Strong medical school statistics are what get you through the door or rather prevent your application from making its way to the recycling bin. Hopefully, you will read this section and have a better understanding of what it takes and if you have potential to pursue a career in medicine.

For the 2020-2021 application cycle there was over 53,000 applicants but only a little over 22,000 matriculated. In other words, only 42% of the applicant pool made it into medical school. Some programs are obviously more competitive than others and this individual data can be found online through each respective medical school's website or through the paid Medical School Admission Requirements (MSAR) platform. We will review the MSAR in the future so do not go running off spending money prematurely. As you can see getting into medical school is no easy task.

The two most important medical school statistics are your Medical College Admissions Test (MCAT) Score and your Undergraduate Grade Point Average (GPA). Some medical schools refer to this as your cumulative GPA (cGPA). Your GPA can also be further subdivided into your BCPM GPA which stands for Biology, Chemistry, Physics, and Math courses. I will often refer to this GPA as your Science GPA (sGPA). This is calculated when you input all your courses into the American Medical College Application Service (AMCAS).

You can also calculate it yourself using MedicalSchoolHQ GPA Calculator. I would encourage you to do this since your overall GPA you get from your pharmacy program is not equivalent to your sGPA. As a pharmacy student you will find that you will have taken far more credits that count towards your sGPA than traditional applicants. You are spending two extra years in school so adding more grades can be beneficial to minimize a few B's and C's along the way. Medical schools appreciate a high cGPA but take more interest in a strong sGPA. The sGPA demonstrates proficiency in courses related to science and medicine, which admissions feel is a more accurate predictor of future academic success considering our line of work. In general, its far easier to get an "A+" in "English 101" than it is to get the equivalent grade in "Organic Chemistry 202." Your sGPA reflects this reality and it holds more weight in the eyes of an admission officer. This process may seem trivial, but it can give you a good idea of where you stand.

I have listed some important statistics from the most recent application cycle below for your reference. You can use these statistics to gauge how qualified you are to apply to medical school. We will discuss the complexities of a strong application in more depth in later sections. Alas do not get discouraged if you fall below these averages. Plenty of students get in with subpar statistics and I can almost guarantee you that none of them have pharmacy doctorates.

2020-2021 Application Cycle:

Average MCAT (Allopathic):	511.5
Average MCAT (Osteopathic):	503.8
Cumulative GPA (Allopathic):	3.73
Cumulative GPA (Osteopathic):	3.54
sGPA (BCPM):	3.66
Non-Science GPA:	3.82

CALCULATE YOUR LizzyM SCORE:

The **LizzyM Score** is used to quantify your chances of getting into medical school using the success rates of other applicants with similar medical school statistics. You can use this tool to determine the odds of getting accepted based solely on your GPA and MCAT scores. This can be a useful tool to give you a snapshot of your application health, but the calculator neglects other facets of a strong application. Also, just because the calculator says you have a "75% chance of getting accepted somewhere" does not mean you will be part of that cohort. You could very well be part of the 25% with the same stats that did not get in. Use this tool to get a rough idea of where you stand but do not rely on it beyond that. Check out the calculator through the link or QR code below.

TAKEAWAYS:

- Statistically speaking, only 42% of applicants will ever matriculate.

- Receiving a medical school acceptance is getting harder every year.

- A strong MCAT and GPA are essential to a strong application.

- Your sGPA is more valuable than your cGPA.

- The LizzyM Score can be a useful metric to determine your percent chance of getting an acceptance.

EXTERNAL RESOURCES:

- **Resource:** Medical School HQ GPA Calculator
  https://medicalschoolhq.net/med-school-gpa-calculator-for-amcas-aacomas-and-tmdsas/

- **Resource:** LizzyM Score Calculator
  https://www.studentdoctor.net/schools/lizzym-score

2. APPLYING TO MEDICAL SCHOOL IS EXPENSIVE:

Although every applicant's experience will be different the financial burden of applying to medical school is often a shared experience. Regardless of your upbringing it is important to recognize that applying is not a cost-free endeavor. As a pharmacy student you will likely already have a substantial amount of debt. According to The American Association of Colleges of Pharmacy's 2017 Graduate Student Report, the average graduating pharmacy student will have amassed $163,496 in student loan burden. The scariest part is that this data is from 2017 and the loan burden is likely even higher today. I myself graduated pharmacy school owing approximately $150,000, slightly below the national average. Regardless, mortgage sized education loans are no laughing matter. This is not to scare you away from pursuing a career in medicine but rather to provide some perspective. Assuming you have a considerable student loan burden like I do, deciding to continue your education warrants a financial inspection. You now have a fiduciary responsibility to yourself to protect your finances more so than ever before.

It is not an easy task convincing your family, loved ones, professors, and peers that you are going back to school. Some may even think you are crazy! That six-figure pharmacist salary that is almost guaranteed at the end of your schooling will fall to the wayside to take on even greater debt. This is no easy decision, and I am only talking about the financial implications at the moment. This life-altering decision has many other complexities that you the reader must wrestle with individually. You must be willing to add years to your schooling experience, handle the mental burden of new information, and now complete a residency after graduating with your medical doctorate. This career shift also has many appealing attributes, otherwise you wouldn't be reading this book. This transition isn't for every pharmacy graduate but those who are considering this route need to limit their expenses to the best of their ability during the application cycle and throughout medical school.

Disregarding your future medical school tuition, the application process itself can be very expensive. These expenses can balloon if you are not careful but also do not try to cut corners to save a few dollars. I would much rather be a broke medical student than to save a few dollars on the front-end only to end up reapplying the following year. This is not to encourage you to blow out the budget but for you to understand a few extra thousand dollars upfront is far better than not becoming an attending physician ten years later. For example, when I first took the MCAT I elected to utilize free resources only. I believed that my pharmacy school education was sufficient to excel on the exam. Well, I could not have been further from the truth. It ended up costing me far more later on when I needed to enroll in a prep-course, re-purchase the MCAT, and invest thousands of hours into preparation. Do not try to cut corners!

As a pharmacy student it may be difficult to scrape up a few thousand dollars for applications. If you are a practicing pharmacist theses costs will sting but won't dramatically impact your net worth. For students, save up all your birthday money, pick up a few extra shifts at your local pharmacy, or take out a few extra thousand dollars on your school loans. You can certainly be frugal throughout the process but the last stressor you need is a financial one.

PHARM.D. TO M.D.

For your reference I have listed some cost you will encounter on the application trail. This process takes more than it gives but getting that acceptance letter makes it all worth it in the end, believe me! Of course, it is impossible to accurately predict every little cost along the way and each student's experience will be unique. Please note that the costs are always rising so if you are budgeting, always compensate for a little over-charge. The chart below is far from comprehensive, but I hope it will provide you with a rough idea of what you are up against.

Investment Contribution	Minimalist ($)	Average ($$)	House in the Hamptons ($$$)
MCAT Cost	$320		
Test Prep	Free Resources Only	AMCAS Material ($500)	Test Prep Course (>$1,500)
CASPER (Altus Suite)	$12 for Test $12 x # of Programs Ex.) 15 programs = **$192**	20 programs = **$252**	25 programs = **$312**
Primary Application	$170 for 1st School $42 for extra schools Ex.) 15 programs = **$800**	20 programs = **$968**	25 programs = **$1,178**
MSAR	$28		
Secondary Applications	$100 per school Ex.) 15 programs = **$1,500**	20 programs = **$2,000**	25 programs = **$2,500**
Interview Travel	Highly dependent on the number of interviews you receive and how far away they are. (~$2,000)		
M.D. Deposits	~$100 and refundable		
D.O. Deposits	~$1,000 per school and NON-refundable		
Total	**$5,940**	**$7,168**	**$8,938**

From my personal experience, I ended up spending closer to $10,000 after everything was said and done. To be fair, I was neither the smartest nor the most strategic during my application cycle. I applied very broadly to over 33 programs (yikes!). Within my large program list, I failed to adequately review school specific application requirements and had to forgo my pursuit of acceptance along with any associated financials. For example, I was overzealous when applying to reach programs, and unrealistic about getting into programs with severe in-state biases. I tossed away hundreds of dollars in poorly coordinated primary applications and took a bare minimum approach to MCAT preparation which resulted in a costly retake.

While the final result was a medical school acceptance, the manner in which I did it was far from strategic and even less coordinated than I would have hoped. We will address some of these important shortcomings and how to keep your balance sheet out of the red. Check out Medical School Headquarters' **Application Cost Estimator** to calculate your own potential costs. This is a very useful tool and unfortunately, all too realistic.

There are many resources available to you to help limit the cost burden of applying to medical school. We will focus on programs and opportunities that Pharmacy students may find appealing.

#1: The Association of American Medical Colleges (AAMC) can assist applicants through their **"Fee Assistance Program."** Qualifications include demonstrating proof of citizenship and providing parental income values. Check out their **website** to see if you qualify.

#2: Consider applying to an **MD-PhD Program**. This is an extremely competitive application process that allows participants to complete a hybrid education plan. They start off completing the first 2 years of medical school, then 3-4 years for PhD. attainment, followed by the final 2 years of medical school. The incentive to take on this indirect route to becoming a physician includes a cost-free medical school education. The tradeoff for a free education is an additional 3-4 years of your life spent in an academic research lab. You can learn more about this specific program in the "**Additional Resources**" chapter.

#3: The Military's **Health Professions Scholarship Program,** otherwise known as HPSP for short. I bring this up because it is one of the most commonly offered scholarships and its features almost seem too good to be true. In short, the military will pay for all your medical school expenses including tuition and supplies. They also provide the student with a monthly stipend for living expenses. In turn, at the completion of your schooling you are expected to pay back the contribution through equal years of service as a military doctor.

   A career in the military is certainly not for everyone but an offer this attractive is often hard to overlook. As a pharmacy student riddled with debt, I found this program to be extremely appealing, at least at face value. As the old proverb goes, "if it's too good to be true, it probably is." While the upsides of the program are quite obviously marketed by the military, the downsides are often realized much later. I have listed a few Pros and Cons about the program, and you can read through and see if this scholarship opportunity is appropriate for you.

Pros:
1. **Your tuition costs are completely covered.** This "pro" should be weighted considerably more as the cost of your medical school tuition rises. This scholarship will be far more fruitful to the recipient if they attend an out-of-state private institution compared to their public in-state programs.

2. **You will receive a monthly stipend of approximately $2,000 per month.** The monetary value will vary based on your medical school location and your branch of military you intend to serve under.

3. **There is an opportunity for large signing bonuses which can exceed $20,000.** To qualify for these bonuses, you are often required to complete a 4-year service obligation.

4. **You have an opportunity to serve in the American Military and will have access to most, if not all, benefits allocated to military personal.** A career dedicated to the service will provide ample military benefits and open the door for pension eligibility.

5. **You will have the opportunity to travel and see more of the world than any civilian physician would ever have access to.** This feature is highly variable, and I have been told from current physicians in the program that the military attempts to work with you to match your travel requests. This however can also be slotted as a "con." See below for more details.

6. **Lastly, physician residency pay is on average higher than civilian residency pay.** A recent study published in Cureus found that on average military residents earned 53% more than their civilian resident counterparts. This flips dramatically once you become an attending (another major "con" listed below).

Cons:
1. **You may have less autonomy regarding the selection of your future specialty.** The military only needs certain types of physicians, and they will likely put limitations on what you can specialize in. This is related to the number of military residency match positions available each year. The military needs far more emergency medicine and trauma surgeons than they need pediatric oncologists. If you are interested in a very specific subspecialty you may want to investigate the current demand for said profession before signing up for the HPSP.

2. **Although you received payments and tuition coverage upfront, you will have to pay this back through equivalent years of service.** If you accepted a 4-year scholarship, you are expected to pay back those years in service. Another important consideration is that your residency training DOES NOT count towards repayment, even if you participate in the military match. You are also subject to deployments and can be placed wherever the military needs your services at that point in time. This may not always fit with your personal schedule, especially if you are interested in starting a family or your own private practice.

3. **As a military attending, your salary is far lower than a civilian equivalents salary.** According to the same Cureus study the military attending made 32%-58% less than their civilian counterparts. To put this into perspective, consider the numbers. If you are an orthopedic surgeon in the military, your civilian counterpart will make approximately 50% more gross annual income. Instead of the $500,000 attending salary you were expecting, you will only make approximately $250,000. Multiply this deficit by 4 years for repayment purposes and you are short $1,000,000. The opportunity cost of pursuing a career in the military far exceeds any potential benefit you may experience from a cost-free medical education which averages no more than $350,000.

The HPSP scholarship may be attractive at first glance, but it has some drawbacks hidden away in the details. Considering our substantial pharmacy school loan burden this program may help prevent you from succumbing to even more debt, but I hope you understand what you are signing up for. The best advice I can offer is for you to talk with someone who is currently in the program. Their experience and insight will be worth far more than some conjecture in a book.

You can learn more about this program through the on the next page. If you are committed, you should reach out to a military recruiter, and they will facilitate your enrollment!

TAKEAWAYS:

- The average pharmacy graduate has $163,496 in student loan debt.

- Applying to medical school is expensive.

- Apply smartly and you will save money by default.

- AAMC offers a Fee Assistance Program for qualifying applicants.

- The MD-PhD program may be a viable option for students interested in research while covering their education costs.

- You can seek a free medical school education through the HPSP program but read the fine print before signing up.

EXTERNAL RESOURCES:

- **Resource:** Medical School HQ Application Cost Estimator
  https://medicalschoolhq.net/medical-school-applications-cost-estimator/

- **Resource:** AAMC Fee Assistance Program
  https://students-residents.aamc.org/fee-assistance-program/fee-assistance-program

- **Resource:** HPSP Scholarship
  https://www.goarmy.com/amedd/education/hpsp.html

3. CHOOSING A MEDICAL SCPECIALTY:

You may be wondering, "why is this guy talking to me about choosing a specialty right now? All I want to do is know how to get into medical school." I completely understand so I will keep this section short. You will have plenty of time throughout medical school to soul-search and find your true passion. I am introducing this concept because having a general idea upfront can help motivate you throughout the application cycle. Additionally, having a set specialty can help you navigate difficult questions you may receive throughout the interview season. For instance, "I loved pharmacy school, and it helped me identify that I am extremely passionate about pursuing a career in anesthesiology." We will discuss the intricacies of interviewing in future chapters.

Another facet pharmacy graduates need to consider when choosing a specialty in medicine is the opportunity cost of lost income as a pharmacist. Don't worry, this isn't another chapter on finance, but I want to introduce the idea that you should consider your future attending salary. I am not saying you should select your career based on the highest paying position, but it certainly needs to be part of the discussion. A pharmacy graduate is starting medical school sometimes 2-4 years later than most matriculants. That's 2-4 years of attending income you will never see, unless you plan on making up for it by working until you are 70. Pharmacy graduates have high debt burdens, and a higher paying specialty will help remove some of the financial pressure you may face. Lastly, the opportunity cost of attending medical school is much higher for pharmacy graduates than it is for traditional biology graduates.

According to the Bureau of Labor Statistics the median pharmacist pay in 2020 was $128,720. In comparison, graduates with a bachelor's degree only made $48,400 on average. Based on these crude numbers you can extrapolate the forgone income based on your time in medical school and the time you spend completing residency training. Factoring in your future specialties income it will take a pharmacy graduate far longer to overcome the lost income than it will for a biology graduate. Therefore, pharmacy graduates should consider higher paying specialties to offset this financial imbalance.

This is not to say you should avoid family medicine, but it will take you far longer to recover financially. For instance, the 2020 Medscape Family Medicine Physician Compensation Report found that the average compensation was $234,000 a year. When you decide to pursue your medical education, you are throwing away any potential pharmacy income. Factoring in 4 years of medical school and 2 years of residency training you will have forgone 6 years of pharmacy income. That amounts to a total of $772,320 in lost income by going to medical school to become a family physician. The average medical school debt is $215,900. Add this to your pre-existing pharmacy debt (~$163,496) and we are sitting at negative $379,396. I have included the pharmacy loans to this equation because of the inability to begin paying them off due to your education extension. Now add this all together and the opportunity cost of going to medical school is negative $1,151,716. That's over a million dollars that a pharmacy student is behind and that's just for the shortest residency training period. Review the chart below to emphasize how important choosing a specialty really is.

Opportunity Cost of becoming a Family Physician	
Start	-$1,151,716
Year 1	-$917,716
Year 2	-$683,716
Year 3	-$449,716
Year 4	-$215,716
Year 5	**+$18,284**
Notice how it would take 5 years of attending salary ($234,000) just to break even and this calculation is extremely optimistic. I have excluded tax calculations and interest accrued on loans for simplicity. This model also operates under the assumption that your entire income is going towards loans which is extremely unrealistic.	

Now let us use a higher paying specialty to see how the growth compares. The average income for an orthopedic surgeon is $498,080 a year. They must receive at least 5 years of residency training which extends the pharmacy income opportunity cost to a whopping deficit of $1,666,596.

Opportunity Cost of becoming an Orthopedic Surgeon	
Start	-$1,666,596
Year 1	-$1,168,516
Year 2	-$670,436
Year 3	-$172,356
Year 4	*+$325,724*
Year 5	*+$823,804*
Notice how it would take much less time to overcome your debt/opportunity cost. Also, the growth is exponential thereafter.	

Look at the chart below and feel free to crunch your own numbers and see how long it would take to come out positive. Add your anticipated cost of medical school tuition and current pharmacy school debt for an even more accurate prediction. Making more money leads to faster loan repayment but life isn't just about money. I only hope that you take the opportunity cost a pharmacist experiences into consideration when making your decision.

PHARM.D. TO M.D.

Opportunity Cost	Profession Example	Biology Graduate ($48,400 Lost Per Year)	Pharmacist ($128,720 Lost Per Year)
4 Years of Medical School	N/A	$193,600	$514,880
Now choose your anticipated specialty to see the opportunity cost.			
2 Years of Residency	-Family Medicine	$96,800	$257,440
3 Years of Residency	-Emergency Medicine -Internal Medicine	$145,200	$386,160
4 Years of Residency	-Radiologist -Anesthesiology	$196,600	$514,880
5 Years of Residency	-General Surgery	$242,000	$643,600
1-2 Year Fellowship	-Orthopedic Surgeon -Trauma Surgeon -Transplant Surgeon	$290,400	$772,320
7 Years of Residency	-Neurosurgery	$338,800	$901,040

At this point you are probably wondering if I am even an advocate for pharmacy students going into medicine? We aren't even 40 pages into this book, and you are probably reconsidering even applying. Believe me when I say this but **going to medical school was the best decision I ever made!** Even when factoring the financials and extra years of schooling I have no regrets. Do not let these first couple sections discourage you! You are also probably wondering when I am going to start discussing how to apply. Hang tight, in the next section we will begin to discuss the principles of applying and what to expect.

TAKEAWAYS:

- Choose a medical specialty that you are passionate about.

- If you enjoy two different specialties equally, choose the one that pays more.

- Be aware of the pharmacy income opportunity costs and understand that these downside costs impact pharmacists more because of their forgone six-figure income.

4. MAKE AN AAMC ACCOUNT:

Congrats on making to the first active portion of this book. You survived the finance section so applying should be easy right? I do not think we are quite there yet, but the first step is to make an **AAMC Account**. The AAMC website will serve as your conduit to the medical world. On this website you will have access to a plethora of resources, many of which I will discuss in this book. Creating an account now is strongly encouraged, and necessary when you start to apply. When doing so make sure you use a personal email and not a university affiliated account. Depending on your institution, you may lose access to your university email upon graduation. I found it useful to create a whole new email to keep my medical school emails and affairs organized. When you are applying, AMCAS (the application portal) will utilize the same email information. That's it, short and sweet. Off to the next section!

- **Resource:** AAMC Create Account Page
  https://www.aamc.org/

5. REACH OUT TO YOUR UNIVERSITY'S PRE-HEALH ADVISORS:

This section only applies to students who are currently in pharmacy school or enrolled in a university. Graduated pharmacists can skip this section as you will likely not have access to campus resources anymore.

While in pharmacy school I had the opportunity to enroll with my university's pre-health program. I had reached out to several of the advisors in the program explaining my interest in pursuing medical school after pharmacy school. They recommended that I participate in the program, and by doing so I would have access to traditional pre-medical student resources. This would include personal mentoring, general guidance, and networking with other pre-health students. If you have access to this then I encourage you to explore this opportunity, especially since you will be able to receive a committee letter. This letter, although not essential, is very helpful to have and helps you avoid yet another application pitfall.

Unfortunately, I never got around to enrolling in the program because of the added tuition costs and the additional responsibilities. I applied without the support of the university and subsequently lacked a committee letter. Not having said letter did prevent me from getting into some programs who believed that my application was left incomplete. For those of you who do not wish to enroll I would still establish a line of contact with the pre-health office who may be able to assist in application questions or give you a rough idea of how "healthy" your application is. Remember, these advisors do this for a living so having insider tips can go a long way!

6. TAKE THE MCAT FIRST AND TAKE IT SERIOUSLY:

Now that you have created your AAMC account and have established a line of contact with your university's pre-health, we can begin to discuss the most important step for getting into medical school, the MCAT. Performing well on the MCAT (Medical College Admission Test) is by far the most challenging part of the entire application cycle. Getting accepted to a medical school program is highly dependent on having a good score. This test is not the only factor that is considered when applying but it serves as a rate limiting step, a reference to all those chemistry fans out there.

We will discuss the MCAT in great detail in **PART THREE**, but I am introducing this here to emphasize how important this exam is. Do not take it lightly. Please do not make the mistake of believing your pharmacy background will have adequately prepared you for this monstrous exam. It requires extensive preparation including content mastery and an understanding of specific test taking strategies. I personally underestimated this exam and subsequently scored in the 38th percentile, which led to a retake. Scheduling another MCAT attempt complicated my application cycle and added another 4 months of preparation to my already busy schedule.

As a pharmacy student my recommendation to you is to take this exam during the summer between professional year 2 (PY2) and professional year 3 (PY3). This will leave you ample time for a retake if required, and if not, plenty of time to build a strong medical school application.

If you are a younger pharmacy student reading this book, you may be able to take it between your PY1 and PY2 years. This may afford you more time for potential retakes, but you run the risk of having your exam score expire. Your MCAT score is only valid for 3 years after completion of the exam. In other words, you will need to receive an acceptance to a program within that time window, or you will need to retake the MCAT, despite having a good score. That means during your PY4 year of school while applying!

If you are an older pharmacy student in their PY3 year or beyond (including graduates), take the MCAT when your schedule permits. This is ideally when you have limited distractions from work and/or exams. I was forced to take my MCAT during my second semester of PY3 year right before the application cycle opened. It is certainly possible to achieve this but preparing for the MCAT during this period of my life was extremely stressful and took away from bettering my application. If you are a rising PY3 student or PY4 take the exam during scheduled rotation off-blocks. Pharmacy graduates will need to consider taking time off from work or remain disciplined to study after your shifts.

I recommend that you take the MCAT first before committing time to improving your application. Your MCAT score is a major component to getting into medical school and a subpar score will hold you back. I would hate for you to throw your heart and soul into creating the perfect application but having a bad MCAT score holding you down. We will discuss what makes a good application in future sections so do not worry about that here. As I mentioned the MCAT will make or break your application so dedicate all your time and effort to this **First**.

7. YOUR PHARM.D. IS YOUR MOST PRIZED POCESSION:

Very few medical school applicants will have such a unique educational background so use it to your advantage when applying. I found it relatively easy reflecting on clinical patient interactions when writing my primary application and it was due to our high quantity of pharmacy rotations. You will find interviews very enjoyable as well. It is the first face-to-face opportunity to truly demonstrate that you are a healthcare professional. The interview will feel natural to you and as if you are talking to just another physician on the hospital ward. Pharmacy school not only teaches you the intricacies of pharmacy, but it fosters a sense of professionalism that sets you apart on interview day. However, don't be fooled into thinking you are the strongest applicant in the room. You will interview with a diverse crowd of students who each have unique experiences, research achievements, etc. They will all be trying to put forward their best self. I am only encouraging you to do the same!

I have placed this section here for you to really consider the "million-dollar question" (literally): **"Why medicine and why not pharmacy?"** You will need to have a strong, logical, and concise answer to this defining question. Everyone you encounter – ranging from the physician conducting your interview to the barista at the hospital coffee shop – will look at you as if you are crazy. Convince them that you want to be there and that you are ready for the next chapter of your life!

I have also placed this section here to emphasize that **your PharmD is unique, but it will not push you through**. We will address how to create a holistic application later but keep this critical statement in your mind. The next part will introduce a schedule which you can follow at your leisure in order to maximize your chances of getting into medical school.

PHARM.D. TO M.D.

PART TWO:

THE SCHEDULE

"To study the phenomena of disease without books is to sail an uncharted sea, while to study books without patients is not to go to sea at all."

– William Osler

In this section, we will dive into each Professional Year of Pharmacy school and create a framework for you to follow as you progress through your schooling. When I was busy studying for pharmacy school exams and completing clinical rotations, I hardly had time to get organized. I have created an abbreviated list for you to review below. Feel free to jump to the section that best suits your current year in school. I would encourage you to read over each section to ensure that you do not miss any critical steps along the way. If you are a graduate already, this section will serve as a checklist, and not so much as a template of action. You will still have to complete the application requirements but at your own individualized pace.

PHARM.D. TO M.D.

1. **UNDERGRADUATE YEARS:**

2. **PROFESSIONAL YEAR ONE (PY1):**
    a. Get involved in research opportunities:
    b. Create an AAMC Account:
    c. Start Shadowing Physicians:

3. **PROFESSIONAL YEAR TWO (PY2):**
    a. Complete a medical mission trip:
    b. Take the MCAT:
    c. Continue to shadow physicians and complete research:
    d. Have you taken the correct prerequisites:

4. **PROFESSIONAL YEAR THREE (PY3):**
    a. MCAT Round Two:
    b. Letter of Recommendation:
    c. Draft Your Personal Statement and Work Experiences For AMCAS:
    d. Advanced Practice Pharmacy Experience (APPE) Rotations:
    e. Do not forget to budget:
    f. Determine if the Early Decision Program is right for you:
    g. Complete the Primary Application through AMCAS:
    h. Complete Secondary Applications:

5. **PROFESSIONAL YEAR FOUR (PY4):**
    a. Take the CASPER Exam:
    b. Interview Time:
    c. Provide Update Letters to Programs:
    d. Letter of Intent:
    e. Seeking Pharmacy Licensure (NAPLEX and MPJE):

6. **LICENSED PHARMACIST:**
    a. See Above:

Use this schedule as a generalized framework to guide you throughout pharmacy school and gauge your application health. For instance, if you are a PY4 student but have no research experience and hardly any shadowing hours, your application is far from complete. In comparison if you are a PY1 reading this book and follow these steps algorithmically, you will be very well prepared. Unfortunately, the medical school revelation many pharmacy students encounter often presents itself during the back end of our schooling (PY3 and PY4 years). With that said, try to fit in as much as you can in with the time you have. It is important that you do not rush your application though. If you plan on applying, make sure it's a representation of your best self. Second time applicants struggle far more than first timers!

Note: This schedule is designed for students who wish to matriculate directly from pharmacy school into medical school. If you are planning on a gap year you will have even more time to perfect your application!

UNDERGRADUATE YEARS:

If you are an undergraduate, consider switching to a premedical track. The pharmacy route is far more difficult and expensive! Students in the professional phase of pharmacy school are likely committed to the pharmacy path due to the inability to transfer pharmacy specific credits. In other words, **this is your last chance to reconsider a career in pharmacy**! There are much easier ways to get into medical school. Trust me!

PROFESSIONAL YEAR ONE (PY1):

During your PY1 year you are likely still adjusting to the heavy course load and professional responsibility thrust upon you. Pharmacy school, just like medical school, expects far more from you than any undergraduate curriculum. This year should be dedicated to adjusting to the rigors of pharmacy school and achieving excellent academic performance. If you find yourself in good shape academically, you can start planning out your medical school approach.

GET INVOLVED IN RESEARCH OPPORTUNITIES:

Having a strong research background is a fundamental component to a holistic medical school application. The more years of experience you the more likely you are to get publications and presentations. Medical schools love seeing applicants who are dedicated to advancing medicine, and conducting academic research is the primary conduit to do so.

Pharmacy school faculty always have projects available so do not hesitate to send out a few emails. It never hurts to ask and doing so can facilitate faculty networking that will last for many years to come. If a project isn't readily available, the professor will have your contact information and you will be more likely to get projects in the future.

You should also consider applying to undergraduate research programs that you can complete over the summer. These tend to offer financial compensation for your work which is always appreciated. Most programs also allow you to continue your project past the end of the summer which can turn short-term projects into longitudinal research works.

Despite the positive attributes related to conducting research, I recommend you take on research projects that you are passionate about. Conducting research can be time-consuming, tedious, and downright difficult. These factors can magnify if the project you are working on is of no interest to you! You may not have the luxury to be picky upfront about research opportunities, but you are far more likely to continue your work over the years if you are passionate about it!

MAKE AN AMCAS ACCOUNT:

The American Medical College Application Service (AMCAS) platform is where you will spend the majority of your time during the application cycle. Create an account to familiarize yourself with the platform. However, creating an account does not mean you should start filling out your application. This is just for learning purposes. You should be focusing on bolstering your application and getting good grades in pharmacy school at this point in time.

START SHADOWING PHYSICIANS:

You might not have direct access to physicians at this point in your pharmacy training but it's never too early to get some exposure. Reach out to family friends or relatives in the healthcare field who may be able to put you in contact with practicing physicians. Your Pharmacy faculty can also be a resource but be prepared to defend your interests. As long as you are honest, many faculty mentors would be happy to connect you with one of their attending co-workers.

If you are like me and have no healthcare professionals within your family circle, you may want to start with shadowing clinical pharmacists. This will help introduce you to the hospital policies, broaden your understanding of pharmacist responsibilities, and allow you to network with residents and attendings. Working with a practicing pharmacist will have you understand if you will be happy following through with your education or if you need to make the switch.

The more physician shadowing hours you have under your belt the more validated your transition will appear to application reviewers. What better way to justify your transition out of pharmacy than by having thousands of hours of shadowing experience to back you up!

PROFESSIONAL YEAR TWO (PY2):

Now that you have a year of pharmacy under your belt you should have pretty good time management skills. It is now time to start developing your medical school portfolio. PY2 year affords its own challenges, such as more challenging courses and the opportunity to take on leadership roles in clubs/organizations. The clinical courses you take during this year are what convinced me to pursue a career in medicine. Enjoy them!

COMPLETE A MEDICAL MISSION TRIP:

Spring break is an excellent time to complete a weeklong global health experience. Look into your universities study abroad office and see if they offer any medical mission trips. Most university's will be affiliated with organizations that give students the opportunity to volunteer their time for international service initiatives. The trip may not be medically related, but I can promise you the experience will certainly be worthwhile. The pharmacy curriculum is fairly rigid, and students traditionally struggle to find time to study abroad. You may not be able to spend a semester in Europe but a trip over a short break or during your summer should suffice. If you are unable to find a trip through your university, you can either propose a trip to pharmacy faculty or investigate various third-party coordinators. There are many philanthropic organizations online but the most referenced is "Doctors Without Borders." Full disclosure: I completed a medical mission trip through my university so I cannot speak from experience concerning these online resources. Do your own research and determine what the best option may be for you.

Completing a medical mission trip provides you with an opportunity for hands on clinical experience, while fostering individual character development. You will certainly not regret this opportunity, and it demonstrates that you are committed to helping those in need. Experiences like these make for a unique application!

One major drawback to completing a medical mission trip is the cost. Depending on where you go and the time of the year some trips may exceed $3,000. Budget accordingly and find affordable programs. If international travel is not within your financial means, you can also consider local community mission work. There are plenty of underserved populations lacking adequate medical care in rural and urban parts of the United States.

TAKE THE MCAT:

The summer after your PY2 year is the perfect time for your first MCAT attempt. I will discuss this exam in more depth in the next chapter of this book so do not get bogged down here. In general, I recommend that you start studying after your spring finals and plan to take the exam right before your PY3 fall semester begins. Sacrificing your summer may not seem too appealing upfront but it will give you ample time for a retake if necessary.

If you take the exam any sooner, you run the risk of having your score expire. The MCAT score is only valid for 3 years and some medical school programs only accept scores within 2 years.

CONTINUE TO SHADOW PHYSICIANS AND COMPLETE RESEARCH:

Medical schools love to see continuity. This also allows you to gather more hours and follow through with research projects that can take years to complete. While it is nice to get a variety of experiences from different shadowing offices, it will be most valuable to get several hundred hours form a singular office, as opposed to only get 15 hours from 3 different offices. While variety in experience is important the quantity of hours is far more valuable.

PHARM.D. TO M.D.

HAVE YOU TAKEN THE CORRECT PREREQUISITES?

According to AAMC, medical school programs require 8 Credits of Introductory Biology with lab, 8 credits of English, 8 credits of General Chemistry with lab, and 8 credits of Organic Chemistry with lab. This list is considered an absolute minimum requirement and almost all programs demand additional prerequisites. These would include, but are not limited to, 4 credits of Biochemistry, 8 credits of physics with lab, 8 credits of mathematics. I have listed this information in a table below for easier viewing purposes. Read through the chart and make sure you have passed all these courses and have completed the mandatory credit amount. For reference, 4 credits are equivalent to one semester, while 8 credits equate to two semesters worth.

Course Title	Credit Requirement
General Biology I & II with Labs	8
English with Writing	6-8
General Chemistry I & II with labs	8
Organic Chemistry I & II with labs	8
Biochemistry (Lab not required)	4
Physics I & II with labs	8
Mathematics (Calculus, Statistics, etc.)	6-8

Fortunately for most pharmacy students, these course requirements are usually fulfilled as an undergraduate. I had all my credits accounted for except for Physics II (4 credits). Depending on your individual pharmacy school curriculum you may have the opportunity to take elective courses in your PY3 year. This is an excellent time to complete any missing prerequisite course work. If you have been following my schedule you will have already completed your MCAT and will be more confident enrolling in extra courses knowing you have a rock-solid MCAT score.

FINANCIAL PRO-TIP: If your pharmacy curriculum allows you to take elective credits you may want to consider taking them at a cheaper university. For instance, during my tenure in pharmacy school I was allotted 9 elective credits. I had the opportunity to take any course offered at the university but unbeknownst to many of my peers, undergraduate level courses were billed at the higher pharmacy credit hour rate. In other words, cheap undergraduate level courses were being pro-rated to match the much higher pharmacy credit billing cost. To better illustrate this, the current rate for a pharmacy credit at my alma mater is $1,723. If you recall, I still needed to take a physics II class to complete my medical school prerequisite requirements. The course itself was a total of 4 credits including a lab section. If I had taken it through my university, those credits would have been billed at the pharmacy credit rate and NOT at the appropriate undergraduate rate. I would have owed $6,892. Alternatively, I enrolled at a local 4-year institution and took an eligible physics II class that only cost me $3,540. I was able to transfer those outside credits into my alma mater to fulfill my pharmacy elective credit obligations. Enrolling into a new 4-year university felt tedious at the time, but it was well worth $3,500 in savings. Check with your pharmacy school advisors and university registrar to ensure that you are eligible for this type of financial maneuver. Remember, it never hurts to ask!

Lastly, if you are unsure whether or not you have met the prerequisite requirements for a particular medical school, don't hesitate to contact the respective program to clarify. They are often willing to work with you and can clarify any ambiguities.

PROFESSIONAL YEAR THREE (PY3):

MCAT ROUND TWO:

Hopefully, this step is long behind you and a retake is not necessary. However, accidents happen and sometimes you need to try again. I had to take the exam twice and you may as well. There is no shame in that. Do not get discouraged, and do not let anybody tell you to give up. As Thomas Watson, former president of IBM once said, "If you want to succeed, double your failure rate." There will be hiccups along the path to success so buckle down, analyze your shortcomings, and fine-tune your approach. PY3 is a great year to try again and will allow you to still matriculate into medical school the same year you graduate pharmacy school.

LETTERS OF RECOMMENDATION:

Select your candidates. Find faculty, employers, research associates, and physicians who are willing to write you a "positive" letter of recommendation. I have placed emphasis on positive because nothing sinks an application like a lukewarm or, dare I say, negative letter of recommendation.

It is important to request your letters early so that a less than ambitious letter writer does not delay your application submission. Start asking in January of your PY3. Have them complete the letters by March. This should give you plenty of time to process the letters and submit them into the Primary Application via AMCAS. Remember, if you are planning to immediately matriculate after graduation you will have to submit your application in the summer during the start of your PY4 year. Medical school applications are submitted almost an entire year in advance.

Make sure you find a physician to write you a letter. If you are planning on applying to osteopathic programs also known as "DO schools," make sure you also get a letter of recommendation from an osteopathic physician. Certain DO programs will require a DO letter of recommendation. Without one, your application will find its way to the recycling bin. Researching which schools require them will not only save you time but money as well.

AAMC developed a short document to guide letter-writers on how to create solid letters of recommendation. I recommend you attach this document in your future email to make the process easier. Your professors, mentors, and supervisors are always busy so try to make writing a letter of recommendation as painless as possible for them. Review the Letters of Recommendation Section in **PART FOUR** for a detailed look into the process.

- **Resource:** AAMC Letter Writing Guidelines https://www.aamc.org/system/files?file=2019-09/lettersguidelinesbrochure.pdf

DRAFT YOUR PERSONAL STATEMENT AND WORK EXPERIENCES FOR AMCAS:

The sooner you create these the less crunched for time you will be. You will not want to delay your application cycle because you developed writers-block. This can be a very time-consuming portion of the application cycle and the more time you have to articulate your experiences the better they will turn out. This is an incredibly tedious process that warrants frequent re-wording and grammar adjustments. Your goal should be to tell your story, extract meaning from past experiences, and most importantly, provide application reviewers with a first glance at who you really are. The late Will Rogers famously said, "you never get a second chance to make a first impression." Show your future readers what you are about!

In short, you will have the opportunity to share 15 experiences and the ability to designate 3 of which are most meaningful. You are limited to 700 characters for ordinary experiences and 1,325 characters for those you designate "most meaningful." Check out PART FOUR: The Primary Application, under the **Work/Activities section** for more details about how and what to pre-write.

ADVANCED PRACTICE PHARMACY EXPERICNE (APPE) ROTATIONS:

As your final months of the didactic portion of pharmacy school come to an end, you will be tasked with picking your PY4 APPE Rotations. I would recommend that you pick rotations that will not overburden you, especially during your application phase. This would include your summer months when you will finalize your primary application and begin to submit secondary applications. The last thing you want is to spend 10 hours a day in a hospital on a challenging rotation and then having to stay up all night working on time-sensitive applications.

I would recommend that you DO NOT complete particularly challenging rotations during your PY4 year unless you have a true passion for the preceptor or line of work. You may find yourself already accepted to a medical school by early October so your focus at this time should be on changing professions, not on fulfilling arduous rotation requirements. Moreover, some rotations may be structured like a miniature pharmacy residency, a career path you are no longer pursuing. These challenging rotations will certainly improve your clinical skills, but they may also grind you down. You are on the horizon of committing yourself to a decade of higher education. Cut yourself some slack and enjoy your final months of pharmacy school.

Some pharmacy schools offer "off-blocks", and I would encourage you to take at least one during this busy summer. If you must complete rotations over the summer, try to get easier rotations with reasonable preceptors. It would be in your best interest to fulfill your community pharmacy requirement or an ambulatory care rotation during this period due to the reasonable work hours.

The interview portion of the cycle begins from early September to the end of March. It will be impossible for rotations and interviews to not conflict, but most preceptors are willing to work with you. You may not have any interviews scheduled at the start of a rotation but can be asked to attend several by its conclusion. I would recommend that you be transparent with your preceptor on your first day and let them know about your post-graduation plans. This will open up a line of communication and allow you to easily coordinate make-up hours for interview absences.

Your stats may help you predict when you will need interview time off as well. For Instance, if you are rocking a 4.0 GPA with a 522 MCAT you should anticipate several interviews in early September and October. If you have a 3.1 GPA and a 502 MCAT, you may not hear from programs until January! There is no perfect tool to predict when you will get interviews but being realistic about your application health can guide you through the cycle. At the end of the day, you will still be a pharmacist so don't sweat the little stuff. You are already on the cusp of a fantastic achievement!

PRO-TIP: Only your first APPE rotation can be used in your Primary Application Work Experiences Section. By the time your Primary Application is due, you may not even have completed a rotation yet. On the application they are looking for completed experiences so the majority of your clinical rotations will not qualify. For instance, when I was accepted to rotations at The Johns Hopkins Hospital and The Cleveland Clinic Main Campus Hospital, I was disappointed when I was not able to mention these prestigious experiences on my applications. When I was picking rotations in my PY3 year, I was under the impression that I would have been able to incorporate these nationally recognized programs into my experiences list. These rotations were challenging and although I have no regrets, I would have certainly enjoyed less responsibility while coordinating medical school interviews.

FINANCIAL PRO-TIP: Elect to take local APPE rotations close to your place of residence. This is another facet of pharmacy school that many university faculty neglect to discuss. They hardly address the financial cost of attending distant rotations. I conducted two out-of-state rotations during my tenure and each one cost more than $1,000 including living expenses. Pharmacy faculty often encourage students to explore different institutions because 99% of the student constituency will select rotations for networking purposes. While broadening your clinical knowledge is important, most of your pharmacy peers will choose a rotation site to gain favor with the institution. Their goal is to pursue future employment or procure a desired residency match position. To them, a distant rotation, and the costs associated with it, are a necessary evil when the upside can involve a potential job offering. While it may be beneficial to make friends in different cities you will have plenty of time to do that while on your future medical school rotations. If your pharmacy school allows it, I would encourage you to move home and complete your APPE requirements at local hospitals and pharmacies. By avoiding apartment rent and distant rotations you could save thousands of dollars and still get great rotation experiences.

DO NOT FORGET TO BUDGET:

I know we have already discussed how expensive the application cycle can be. This is just a friendly reminder to make sure you develop a budget and work a few extra shifts at your pharmacy job. You may even need to take out a few extra thousand dollars in loans. If you are financially constrained but want to add a few more programs to your application list, the last thing you want is to have to wait weeks for a loan approval. You will be surprised how quickly your bank account will drain during the first few months of applications; I promise you that!

DETERMINE IF THE EARLY DECISION PROGRAM IS RIGHT FOR YOU:

The Early Decision Program provides applicants with the ability to submit a singular application to one participating medical school of their choosing. By doing so the student is guaranteed to receive a final decision by October 1st from the institution of choice. If they are accepted, the student is obligated to attend the medical school. They may not apply to other programs and are contractually bound once accepted. If the student is rejected, they are eligible to submit more applications to other medical schools. I have listed a few "Pros" and "Cons" below to help you better understand this path.

<u>Pros</u>:

- **You can apply to your dream school and demonstrate your dedication to the program.** Reasons to do so could include cost-effectiveness, alignment with personal goals, or the school's proximity to family and friends.

- **You will have a final decision by October 1st.** If accepted, your cycle will end, and you can focus your efforts on rotations or begin preparing for pharmacy boards. This can be particularly beneficial if your future medical school is not within the same state as your current pharmacy school – the reason being that you will have plenty of extra time to learn your medical school's state pharmacy laws which will be different than your state specific pharmacy law education.

- **Your application costs are condensed to a singular primary application and secondary application.** This avoids the volume problem that many students face when applying broadly. Taking this path can save you thousands, but don't get swayed by the money. Your future is on the line!

Cons:
- **Electing to complete Early Decision DOES NOT lower the medical school's standards for acceptance.** If you are a mediocre applicant then you will be judged accordingly. In other words, there is no favoritism or preferential treatment for taking this path, compared to a traditional application pathway.

- **There are only a small number of seats allotted to Early Decision Applicants.** This process is highly competitive and is best for unique applicants with standout experiences. Instead of competing for 180 available seats, you are now competing for approximately 10-20. While you may be a pharmacy school graduate, you will still need to have a rock-solid application that fits the particular medical school's metrics.

- **You are contractually bound if accepted so you must be confident that you want to go the program you apply to.** This may not be beneficial if you discover later-on that you don't fit well with the school's mission or its current student population. There are many stories of students dropping out of medical schools due to toxic social environments and a cut-throat student body. Your education is your number one priority but obtaining it without the support of your peers or faculty can be quite awful!

- **A rejection will set you back substantially.** Not only will you have been rejected from your dream school, but you will now have to apply to several new programs very late in the cycle. This is a considerable disadvantage as many programs will have already begun offering interviews or acceptances to regular applicants.

For your full disclosure, I did not participate in the Early Decision Program. To be honest: when I was applying, I did not even know it existed. I cannot speak from experience, but I wanted to cover it to keep you informed about the benefits of this potential application route. Applying to the EDP can be very strategic to qualified individuals but a slight miscalculation on your odds of acceptance can be very detrimental overall. This path is typically reserved for outstanding applicants only, but an outstanding applicant with a pharmacy background will fare even better!

COMPLETE THE PRIMARY APPLICATION THROUGH AMCAS:

AMCAS opens in May but cannot be submitted until June 1st. If you have been following the schedule you should have already pre-written most of the content. All that is left is for you to input your content. Submit your work and await verification. Upon verification completion, your AMCAS application will be sent to each medical school of your choosing. Medical schools will not receive applications prior to July 1st. Completing this portion on time is critical and maximizes your chances of getting into a medical school. I am serious, don't submit this late! **PART FOUR** of this book is devoted to the Primary Application, where we will cover more specifics.

COMPLETE SECONDARY APPLICATIONS:

You will begin to receive secondary applications from early July all the way up until December. Most medical schools will review your primary application and subsequently send you a "secondary application" with additional essays you will need to complete. Historically speaking, secondaries were only sent to qualified applicants who had a good chance of getting into the program. Unfortunately, most medical schools today will automatically send a secondary to every applicant who submitted a primary application to their program. Sorry to disappoint but getting a secondary application from a medical school doesn't make you special.

There are still some programs out there that will reject an applicant even before getting a secondary. These rejections are usually reserved for students who applied to programs well above their means or those who were filtered out due to a low MCAT or GPAs. For example, Wake Forest Medical School will not review an application if the applicant does not have a sGPA of 3.2 or higher and a cumulative MCAT score of 502 or higher. This is just one medical school and there are others who have additional requirements. Research each school prior to submitting your primary or you are literally throwing away your time, energy, and capital. For more information about secondary applications, please review **PART FIVE** of this book.

PROFESSIONAL YEAR FOUR (PY4):

TAKE THE CASPER EXAM:

The CASPER Exam is a 90-minute ethics test that attempts to examine an applicant's "people skills" through various situational judgement tests. The test is designed to place you in the middle of different conflicts between two groups of people and tests how you would handle things. There is usually not just one right answer but various ways of handling each conflict.

You are expected to complete the CASPER Exam only for medical schools that require it. There still are several programs that do not utilize CASPER, so you are "off the hook" if you apply to these programs exclusively. For now, just understand that it is another test you will have to take prior to finishing your applications. Fortunately, it is far easier than the MCAT and requires hardly any preparation so do not sweat it!

We will focus more on this exam and some new components designated as Altus Suite. Altus Suite contains the CASPER Exam, SNAPSHOT, and DUET. Please read **PART SIX** for more information about each specific requirement.

INTERVIEW TIME:

Interviews are in my opinion the most exciting part of the application cycle. You can finally showcase the professionalism that has been engrained in you from years of pharmacy school. This is your opportunity to demonstrate those extra years of research and clinical exposure, along with your capacity for interprofessional collaboration (where many of your fellow applicants fall short). This is also a huge achievement to get an interview. Most programs only offer several hundred interviews during the cycle, and you have been lucky enough to secure one. It is at this point that the odds of getting an acceptance have shifted dramatically in your favor. Do not let it get to your head and certainly do not make the mistake of thinking that you are finished! Getting an interview is a major milestone and another step closer to your goal.

You should expect to hear from programs as early as August and as late as April. Each school operates at its own pace and utilizes its own methods for interview selection so don't get caught up in the online drama. For more information about interviewing, check out **PART EIGHT**.

PROVIDE UPDATE LETTERS TO PROGRAMS:

This is your opportunity to highlight any key improvements to your resume since you submitted all your application materials. If you have been following the schedule, you will have completed your secondaries by September and should now be in the waiting phase. You are at the mercy of the medical schools and their will to grant you an interview or an acceptance off the post-interview waitlist. However, this period is not entirely passive, and you can submit an update letter to the programs of your choosing. Do your research and find out what schools on your list accept updates and find out how they accept them. The last thing you want to do is spend time creating a personalized update letter for a program that will reject your efforts.

PHARM.D. TO M.D.

Make sure the content you provide in the update letter is **substantial and of the highest quality,** such as recent publications, an incredible patient experience, or a respectable new position in the hospital. This is a fantastic opportunity for pharmacy students to broadcast their unique APPE rotations and demonstrate the clinical nature of their involvement. As you will see, some APPE rotations will hardly assign responsibility, while others will expect you to fill the role as an active pharmacist. I have been on rotations where I would represent the pharmacy department on rounds by making medication recommendations to the medical team independently. These make for unique stories that the Admissions Committee will love to hear! Your PY4 year also is the time when much of your pharmacy related research will come to fruition. As pharmacy students, many of you will have been working towards presenting your work at the American Society of Health-System Pharmacists (ASHP) Mid-year Clinical Meeting. This showcase for residency and fellowship applicants is a great opportunity for you to present a poster or give a stand-out presentation. This is yet another excellent experience to demonstrate your passion for research and the propagation of medicine, and certainly a worthy addition to your update letter.

Note: Do not send updates until you have given programs a reasonable amount of time to process your application. You do not want to be that applicant who submits an update 20 minutes after completing the same school's secondary. They will wonder why you did not include that information with your recently submitted contents. Doing so can make you look unorganized, and negatively impact your application chances. Unfortunately, I cannot tell you how long that will be because everyone applies at different times, but generally November or December are reasonable times to submit an update. Here are a few examples of when you may consider sending an update letter.

1. If you have interviewed at the program and haven't heard from them in a while or have been placed on a post-interview waitlist.

2. If you have been placed on a Pre-Interview Waitlist, a letter may remind them that you exist and are doing great things.

3. If you have had no updates about the status of your application since you finished your application, an update letter might jolt them to look into your profile.

Lastly, even if you don't have anything substantial to update your medical schools with (unlikely with your APPE Rotations), you should still consider the gesture. Many programs appreciate the act because it demonstrates that the student is still interested in their program. It will also serve as a touchpoint opportunity where you can contact the program again and let them know that you are "extremely excited to hear from them."

We will cover update letters in more depth in **PART NINE**. In that chapter you will find a sample update letter that I utilized during my own cycle for your reference.

LETTER OF INTENT (LOI):

Are you on a post-interview Waitlist? Was the school you interviewed at the program of your dreams? Is it the only school you have heard from and really need to get in? If you said yes to any of these questions, then you should consider writing a letter of Intent (LOI). This is a document you can submit that allows you to express your profound interest in the specific program and make a pledge to attend said program if accepted. Sound familiar? If you were thinking of the Early Decision Program, then you would be correct. The main differences are that a LOI is much less formal, and you are under no obligation to carry out your pledge. I recommend that if you choose to write one of these letters that it is consistent with your pledge, but I also understand that circumstances can change at a moment's notice. For more information, please review **PART NINE**.

SEEKING PHARMACY LICENSURE (NAPLEX AND MPJE):

Now that you have been accepted to a medical school you can take a breather. You have achieved the ultimate goal and you will one day be a physician. The only question that is left unanswered at this moment is "are you going to be a pharmacist?" Once you have committed to a school you will need to decide if you are going to sit for your boards. Personally, I think it would be a disservice to yourself if you decided to pass them up! You have worked so hard over the years to finish pharmacy school that putting in a few extra months to get your license is but a small feat. The summer after you graduate is by far the best time to seek licensure. You will never have as much free time as you do now and dedicating a few hours to your boards will pay off 10-fold.

Alright, I'll get off my soap box and give you the insider tips. Preparing for the NAPLEX and MPJE are both expensive and a logistical nightmare, especially if your future medical school forces you to cross state borders. The major benefit of studying for the exams (especially the NAPLEX) is that it will help with your medical school journey. I understand that dedicating time to study and prepare can be difficult, especially since you are now on the horizon of starting four more years of intense schooling. In the end, I believe it is still worth it! You will one day have to ask yourself the same question and see where it takes you.

By getting your license, you can also work throughout medical school. Working during this busy period of your life is very uncommon but it will provide you with experience that can help bolster your resume – not to mention the nice chunk of cash you receive working for ~$50/hour. Working a few hours, a week won't pay off your student loans, but it can minimize future expenses. I am currently working as a pharmacist on the side, and it has supported my daily living!

PART THREE:

THE MCAT

"I hated every minute of training, but I said, 'Don't quit. Suffer now and live the rest of your life as a champion.'"

– Muhammad Ali

Welcome to the MCAT chapter! I have been alluding to this specific chapter for some time now but for good reason. As I have mentioned previously, the MCAT is the most important examination you will take leading up to medical school. Your performance on this exam is a heavily weighted portion of your application. I am not going to sugar coat it: you will not enjoy this section. Unfortunately, it is far too important to neglect! Additionally, your pharmacy education will do little to help you succeed on this exam. The challenge involves both the volume of content you are expected to know and personal mastery of test-taking strategies. This exam requires you to understand the style of each question and to work diligently through hundreds of questions with great speed. Achieving a high MCAT score is no easy challenge. As a pharmacy student you are no stranger to massive content dumps. We are all too familiar with professors asking you to memorize minute drug facts and dosing information. You will find that the MCAT content is similar in the sense that you are expected to understand a large chunk of information. The catch is that you are then expected to apply your understanding of the material to new or related situations and answer subsequent questions. However, learning the MCAT material itself, although critical, is not where a top-percentile score comes from. You must focus your efforts on test taking speed, time-management, and critical thinking skills that surpass basic memorization. In this chapter we will investigate ways for you to maximize your score and organize your test taking schedule.

Before you dive in, check out the Complete **MCAT Essentials** provided by the AAMC. This will help explain some of the packages they offer and describe the different registration zones you fall into during test signup. They provide an updated version every year so use the most recently posted package of information.

Additionally, it would be impossible for me to give you every detail necessary to enroll, prepare, and succeed on this test. People have written entire books on the MCAT and the AAMC diocese is a whopping 47 pages alone. As my disclaimer, this chapter will be far from comprehensive. However, I will do my best to highlight the important factors and give you the perspective you are looking for.

- **Resource:** The MCAT Essentials Addendum 2021
  https://students-residents.aamc.org/media/11711/download

THE PHARMACY STUDENT STRUGGLE:

As a pharmacy student you may find studying the MCAT content is frustrating. I know I did! You will need to forgo your clinically oriented approach to medicine and get back to studying basic biology. All those years spent building your clinical skills and medication proficiency will fall to the wayside as you struggle to relearn even the most basic science topics. You can forget about all your hard learned pharmacokinetics equations, disease related medication recommendations, and side effect profiles to fill your head with reading passages about basic physics or chemistry. **My point being that you are going to have to re-train your brain to think like an undergrad and less like a healthcare professional!**

This is not to suggest that the information is easy, but rather to offer a forewarning that you may be frustrated relearning what was long forgotten from undergrad. It will be difficult reading up on IUPAC nomenclature for organic chemistry molecules after you have already had hands on patient experience on your Introductory Pharmacy Practice Experiences (IPPE). You will find that most of the information tested on the MCAT has no real-world application. At least that's the case when comparing it to your pharmacy-based healthcare courses!

I found it personally challenging to transition out of my clinical mindset. What pharmacy student wants to study basic physics principles when we have spent years learning about pathology and black box warnings? Pretty much nobody! My mind had already been trained to dissect patient cases, recommend therapies for infectious endocarditis or scan medication profiles for complex drug interactions. The MCAT does little to tie in higher concepts and instead focuses on the sheer volume of content that can be tested on. Some of the information you come across may feel unimportant in comparison to your previous studies. If your test preparation book focuses on the Krebs Cycle, then you better learn the Krebs Cycle. I want to assure you that everything presented to you matters for the MCAT, regardless of how trivial the details may seem. *Approach each concept with curiosity and an open mind. Learn each detail as if you never learned it before.* It will make all the difference on test day!

MY MCAT BACKGROUND:

You are also probably wondering how I performed on the MCAT myself. Why would you even take my advice if you didn't know how I performed? I may have hinted at it already, but I went from a 497 (35th-Percentile) to a 510 (78th-Percentile). Nothing extraordinary by any means! It was a substantial jump for me, but as you know, a 510 is below the average MD matriculant's average of 511.5. I am clearly not an "MCAT guru," nor will I ever claim to be. There are far better test takers than myself! For those of you interested in my section specific breakdown I received a 125/124/125/123 (497) and 127/125/128/130 (510).

Everyone will have the same starting books and content to read but learning the nitty gritty details will be the defining principle. Everyone utilizes test-prep but not everyone approaches it the correct way. In my experience (corroborated by what the applicant community has found), performance on the MCAT is associated with how disciplined you are. It is not so much the quantity of hours spent preparing that leads to success, but rather the angle you take and how efficiently you use your time. While you will still need to put forth 100% of your efforts to succeed, not everyone invests their time and energy into the right places. "Hard work without intelligence creates sweat, not results."

GETTING TO KNOW THE MCAT:

To begin, we need to start with developing an understanding of what the MCAT is all about. This is a 4-section exam with a total of 230 questions on a variety of different content fields including, but not limited to, physics, chemistry, organic chemistry, critical reading, biology, and psychology. The majority of questions are passage-based questions from each section. Every section, except the CARS portion, has 10 passages with 4-6 questions per passage and 15 independent or free-standing questions, totaling at 59 questions. The CARS portion has 9 passages with 5-7 questions per passage with no independent questions. The chart below has been replicated from AAMC's Essentials Guide to show you what your exam day will look like.

Exam Overview		
Section	Question Count	Time Allotted
Test-Day Certification		4 minutes
Tutorial (Optional)		10 minutes
Chemical and Physical Foundations of Biological Systems	59	95 minutes
Break (Optional)		10 minutes
Critical Analysis and Reasoning Skills	53	90 minutes
Mid-exam Break (Optional)		30 minutes
Biological and Biochemical Foundations of Living Systems	59	95 minutes
Break (Optional)		10 minutes
Psychological, Social, and Biological Foundations of Behavior	59	95 minutes
Void Question		3 minutes
End-of-day survey (Optional)		5 minutes
Total Content Time		**6 hours and 15 minutes**
Total "Seated" Time		**7 hours and 30 minutes**

As you can see this is no walk in the park. This is a time-consuming exam that will can be both mentally and emotionally draining. This is not to scare you, as thousands of people succeed every year, but I want you to be well informed! Now that you know how the test is structured, you are probably wondering how it is even scored.

HOW THE MCAT IS SCORED:

Out of the 4 sections you are graded on the number of questions you get correct for each subsection. This is then adjusted and assigned a percentile rank based on all the other students who took that specific exam and how difficult your questions were. Obviously, there are plenty of different MCAT test dates throughout the year and no student takes the exact same exam (unless it's on the same day). They ask different questions, and one test may be much harder than a previous one. The AAMC board adjusts these scores to represent the difficulty of the questions asked. For instance, if you got 42/59 questions on the Biology Section but your friend got a 42/59 the following test week, you may end up with a higher section score if the questions on your exam were determined to be far more difficult.

In one individual section your score could range from a 118 (lowest) to a 132 (highest). In other words, the best score you can possibly obtain would be a 532 and the worst being a 472. Your personal score will be the cumulative value of each subsection and then you will be assigned a percentile rank. Regardless of how you perform, your score will stick with you forever! Even if you retake the exam your original score will also be reported to your Primary Application in AMCAS. As you know, I begrudgingly took the MCAT twice but when it came time for me to apply, I had to submit my 497 along with 510. Keep this in mind and take your preparation seriously. Otherwise, you will have to discuss this noticeable score shortcoming during some secondaries and possibly during interviews. Check out the percentile data for each score report for your reference.

- **Resource:** Summary of MCAT Total Scores
  https://students-residents.aamc.org/media/8356/download

Lastly, it is important to note that your score report will take one month before it is released to you. This is an important distinction for my PY3 Spring MCAT takers. Scheduling your exam right after your PY3 Spring Finals may seem reasonable but I want you to understand that it can delay your primary application timing. You can submit your primary application without having an MCAT score to get in the verification queue, but it can be risky if your exam score is well below acceptable limits. Alternatively, if you wait too long, you are fighting against the clock to get your application pushed out to medical schools. We will discuss the particulars of applying in PART FOUR.

GETTING STARTED:

There are ample resources available to you ranging from summer MCAT bootcamps to free resources on the web. I have compiled several of these resources with some quick information about that I recommend you use. This is far from comprehensive, but it will hopefully set you off in the right direction.

FREE RESOURCES:

#1: To start, "Khan Academy MCAT" is an excellent for resource for mastering content. They have a large array of online videos explaining material. I used it frequently to clarify some of the more difficult concepts. Check out their website and browse the massive amount of video material available to you.

#2: I recommend that you create a "Reddit" account and join the "r/MCAT" community for access to a variety of resources and real time help from others. After accessing the QR code, you can scroll down to find "High Yield MCAT Links" which you can review as you please. Although this is a forum that is relatively unregulated, I still found it amusing and there are plenty of "pro-tips" from recent test takers and those who have had tremendous success. I also found it reassuring to see that there were other people going through this difficult process at the same time. Studying for the MCAT can be a lonely endeavor, especially for a pharmacy student. You can find motivation and support from this online community to conquer this test! Not to send you down a rabbit hole but I have listed a few "Reddit Success Stories" for some inspiration. 500 to 521 in 6 weeks or Top 10 tips from a 526 scorer.

#3: Our next resource is "Nextstep Test Prep," now formally known as "**Blueprint MCAT**." Here you will find several free full-length and half-length practice exams along with plentiful section specific question bundles, also known as "section banks." I recommend that you take one of these practice exams early on to get a better idea of what you are up against. In general, these full-lengths are slightly easier than the real MCAT and can provide you with artificially high scores. You should use Blueprint resources as a confidence booster or as yet another way to familiarize yourself with the testing format. To access the material, you will have to create an account.

#4: Our next resource is the official "AAMC Sample Test." This will be your first true look at what you should expect on your actual test day. This content is provided by the very same people who create and score the real MCAT. When taking this practice test, treat it like the real deal! That means no breaks except for the allotted time, no pausing or googling mid-exam, etc. If you have never taken a practice MCAT before I would not recommend using this resource as your first attempt. It would likely be wasted, especially since you will not have mastered much of the material so early on. If you have not figured it out already, **AAMC provided content is equivalent to preparation gold**. How you perform on the AAMC practice exams is the most accurate predictor of how you will perform on test day. Use these resources wisely and closer to your test date! Fortunately, they do offer several paid practice exams which we will discuss below.

#5: Our next resource is "JackWestin CARS Passages." Create an account and they will provide you with free CARS passages every day. The CARS section of the MCAT can be very challenging for many applicants. It focuses on reading comprehension and requires special critical thinking skills that are uniquely employed in this section alone. Just like a muscle, you will need to train daily to strengthen these skills. In general, you should aim to complete at least one passage a day. As you get closer to your exam date you should increase the number of passages accordingly. When practicing CARS passages it's important to emulate realistic testing conditions. The best way to do this is to time yourself so that you can train your brain to work quickly and efficiently through passages. The CARS section was the hardest section for me personally and I found JackWestin passages to be helpful along the way.

#6: I recommend you utilize Quizlet Flash Cards, especially after you have concluded study preparation for a particular section. These will help you retain vital information that is quickly lost without rehearsal. I found these particularly helpful for the Psychology/Sociology portion considering the content is the closest you will get to pure memorization. This material is created by other students so be cautious when attempting to learn concepts here. It might not always be 100% accurate or up to date!

EXTERNAL RESOURCES:

- **Resource:** Khan Academy MCAT
  https://www.khanacademy.org/test-prep/mcat

- **Resource:** MCAT Reddit Home Page
  https://www.reddit.com/r/Mcat/wiki/index

- **Resource:** "500 to 521 in 6 Weeks," Reddit
  https://www.reddit.com/r/Mcat/comments/6ob0b2/how_i_went_from_500_to_521_in_6_weeks/

- **Resource:** Top 10 Tips from a 526 Scorer" Reddit
  https://www.reddit.com/r/Mcat/comments/7nbnn5/top_10_tips_ama_from_a_526_scorer/

- **Resource:** Blueprint MCAT
  https://blueprintprep.com/mcat/free-resources/free-mcat-practice-bundle

- **Resource:** JackWestin CARS Passages
  https://jackwestin.com/mcat-question-of-the-day

- **Resoruce:** Quizlet Flash Cards
  https://quizlet.com/latest

FREE DOESN'T ALWAYS TRANSLATE TO QUALITY:

This list of free resources is far from exhaustive! I am sure you will have heard of different options from friends or other online outlets. Use what suits your needs! Although free content is always greatly appreciated, in my experience, it falls short when it comes to <u>structure</u>. Of course, these resources give you plenty of material to browse through but most of it is devoid of a set schedule. When I was preparing for my first MCAT exam in the summer between PY2 and PY3, I made it my goal to invest as little money as possible. At the time, I was unwilling to invest in pricy test preparation material especially when the thought of actually getting into medical school seemed so far off. I figured I would try the MCAT out for fun and see where it took me. You already know how that turned out for me.

While I was busy "nickel and diming" my test prep, I was oblivious to how lost I was in the content. It was overwhelming and every day I would shift my focus to a different platform, website, or resource trying to piece together a study plan. For me personally, it was too much of a hassle and I wasted almost as much time finding these resources as I did actually studying them. Perhaps it will be different for you, now that you have a decent head start on a resource list, but everyone will be different. I personally needed some structure to guide me through the process and keep me on track. Just remember the age old saying, "you get what you pay for" – free isn't always the quality you need and may not provide you with the results you would like. The great irony is that being cheap on the front-end cost me more in the long run!

My main point is if you are planning on taking the MCAT, do it right the first time. Don't skimp out on preparation. Use the free resources when possible, but I wouldn't recommend you use them exclusively. Lastly, if you are gearing up for the MCAT, fix your mindset. You aren't doing this for fun, or just trying it out to brag to your pharmacy buddies. This is a major step in a potentially life-altering decision. If you are going to do it, do it right!

PAID RESOURCES:

You are now entering the **Paid** portion for MCAT preparation. I am sure you will have heard of several of the listed paid services since they make a tremendous effort to market to potential applicants. The list is rather extensive including *Altius MCAT Prep Course, Blueprint Online MCAT Prep Course, Examkrackers MCAT, Gold Standard MCAT Prep Course, Magoosh MCAT, Kaplan MCAT Prep, Khan Academy MCAT Prep Course, The Princeton Review MCAT,* and far more. Each one of these programs has many different subdivisions and types of learning plans you can customize to fit your study needs. For instance, you can take on a minimalist approach and purchase the complete MCAT textbook set. Doing so will provide you with the necessary content and allow you to work at your own pace as needed while getting information from a validated source. Alternatively, you can enroll in a summer MCAT bootcamp where all you do is "eat, sleep, and MCAT." MCAT summer camp is a little much in my opinion but to each is their own. I recommend you choose something in the middle that offers some guidance but allows for independent progression. My point is that there are many resources out there and each will have varying degrees of cost which must be weighted by the potential benefits.

KAPLAN AND PRINCETON:

Since I have not utilized more than a handful of these resources, I can only share what worked for me personally. During my first attempt at the MCAT I utilized the complete **Kaplan Textbook set** that I borrowed from a friend. The textbooks were excellent and provided me with the necessary information. The problem was that once again I lacked the proper structure, and practically "crawled" through the material. I needed something more structured that would guide me through the material, something far more involved than passively reading 1,000-page textbooks. Additionally, the books alone don't provide very many practice problems. A major downside to offline preparation packages.

During my second MCAT attempt I enrolled in **The Princeton Review** Self-Paced MCAT prep course. They provided me with the complete textbook set as well as a comprehensive online platform to organize the material. I had access to video content that was well coordinated with the material I was reading from the textbooks. Each section was heavily interconnected to tie key ideas together and bridge the missing gaps. I also had access to full section banks, thousands of practice questions, and 10+ full-length practice exams. This isn't supposed to be a Princeton Review advertisement, but I was thoroughly impressed with the service I received. To be fair, I am confident that what I experienced can be found through any of the other test prep services available to you. Regardless of the service you choose, I would not be where I am today if I hadn't invested a little bit of money into my future. As we have discussed, there are other ways to drive your overhead costs down, or at least avoid substantial losses. The MCAT is not something to come up short on.

AAMC CONTENT IS NON-NEGOTIABLE:

Speaking of additional costs, **all AAMC content is 100% mandatory to purchase.** Unfortunately, there is no getting around this. The AAMC creates each MCAT exam, and they also create test preparation content. It is absolutely necessary that you utilize every bit of content they provide you with, all of which can be found at the AAMC store. Although third-party test prep like the Princeton Review or Kaplan are excellent tools, you will still need to get your hands on the AAMC material. Fortunately, most third-party packages will come with the AAMC content included so check the fine print. The question style, formatting, and level of detail seen in the AAMC preparation content will be very similar to the exam itself. As a general recommendation, you should utilize third-party test prep for several months before your test date but switch to AAMC material when you are approximately a month out.

There is no exact science as to when you should introduce the AAMC material, but it is best to practice with the same style of questions you will see on exam day. You should also reserve the AAMC Full-length exams for this final month of preparation. Your scores on this content are often reflective of your actual test score and are the best predictor of your future performance. In between these exams, practice with AAMC section banks and commit yourself to an extensive review of your past full-lengths. Analyze what you got wrong and inspect how you came to the wrong answer. Doing so can help you avoid costly mistakes on "game day." Check out the comprehensive list put out by AAMC with details on all the products that they offer.

UWORLD AND EXAMKRACKERS:

Another commonly utilized test prep platform is "**UWorld**." They offer an extensive collection of MCAT-style test questions with comprehensive explanations. I did not personally utilize UWorld, but I felt obligated to share it with you considering it has received extensive praise from my fellow medical school peers.

The last reference I will leave you with will be the **ExamKrackers** 101 CARS Passages. I purchased this handy book that had hundreds of difficult CARS passages that challenged me every day. Along with the JackWestin Passages, I utilized this large collection to fine-tune my CARS strategies.

EXTERNAL RESOURCES:

- **Resource:** Kaplan Textbook Set
  https://www.kaptest.com/mcat?gclid=CjwKCAjwruSHBhAtEiwA_qCppnn1DlFACu5emyMrOghpAn1k421TqpNFl0CND7Yil5UN8Zt3lylR6xoC4OkQAvD_BwE&gclsrc=aw.ds

- **Resource:** The Princeton Review
  https://www.princetonreview.com/medical/mcat-test-prep?ceid=newhp-nav

- **Resource:** AAMC Store
  https://store.aamc.org/mcat-prep.html

- **Resource:** AAMC Product Comparison Chart
  http://image.email.aamc.org/lib/fe8e13727c63047f73/m/1/31cca904-534d-4a62-bf29-d4359c322c51.pdf

- **Resource:** UWorld Home Page
  https://www.uworld.com/collegeprep/mcat/mcat.aspx

- **Resource:** ExamKrackers MCAT
  https://examkrackers.com/product/online-mcat-class/?gclid=CjwKCAjwruSHBhAtEiwA_qCppnvJhPZGhExxOlwNW3qM5IxgkvHCx_Ux6CX_K8c9et9Ec94faCa_3RoCeL8QAvD_BwE

BASIC STRATEGY:

As mentioned before, this test is unlike any pharmacy exam you have taken. The variety of content and pace of the test is unique and should be treated as such. I have told other students gearing up for the MCAT to **study content just as much as the test itself.** That's right, you need to study the cadence of the exam, how it flows, and how to optimize your score.

#1: Learn the content first. Practice the content regularly and reinforce previously learned material by taking full-lengths or completing practice questions.

#2: Learn how to approach particular types of questions. By classifying a question type, you will notice that there are different techniques to help limit answer choices and lead you to the best possible answer. Most test-prep companies will explain this in painstaking detail. Also, be ready to combine learned conceptual information to new passage information. This will include information that you have never seen before and you will need to use your critical thinking skills to work through the prompts.

#3: Test taking speed is very difficult to master. Despite knowing every little detail, you are expected to learn, you will still get questions wrong if you don't have enough time to finish each section. Pacing yourself is essential and spending too much time on a passage can ruin your section score. The last thing you want is to forgo answering several easy questions at the end because you spent too much time working through a challenging question early on.

I wish I could provide you with the perfect study plan to conquer this test, but your success is highly dependent on finding out what works for you. For example, I found that rewriting the biology section in a notebook was very useful for my own style of learning. This was a very taxing process but provided me with a strong biology test score. I created formula sheets for physics and general chemistry equations and typed most of the psychology section. I would also recommend completing several CARS passages each day and time yourself so that you become better at quickly processing new information. Third-party preparation courses will do a far better job explaining the intricacies of the exam, but I hope you can use this to get started! Up next, we will take a look at how to develop a schedule and give you some much needed structure to your study plan.

DEVELOP A PLAN:

Preparing for the MCAT is equivalent to a full-time job. You have a limited number of sick-days and are expected to provide results. It is imperative that you remain focused during this grueling experience and know that what you put into it is what you will get out of it! Your time will be limited and as a pharmacy student you need results, especially if you are taking your MCAT during your PY3 year. There is nothing worse than having your exam a couple weeks out and still learning new content. I know this because I went through it. There is far too much to memorize, let alone understand, in such a short period of time. Maintaining a schedule will guarantee adequate preparation and keep things as stress-free as possible. I created a makeshift timeline that you can use as a rough template to ensure you are on track.

4-5 MONTHS OUT:

#1: Consider taking a sample MCAT test. Although not necessary, this will give you a baseline while allowing you to appreciate the stamina required to sit for this exam. This will serve as your first look at the testing format and style of questions you are expected to answer. You will come to the valuable realization that taking the MCAT requires far more than knowledge alone. Don't get discouraged by a "bad" score. This is only the first step on the road to success.

#2: Start your content review by utilizing resources of your choosing. I would recommend a hybrid of a 3rd party course along with the free material I mentioned above. Work through each chapter of the material and focus on one section at a time. This excludes CARS which should be practiced almost every day. As you get closer to your exam date you can gradually increase the number of passages you complete. I personally started with the biology content because it was one of my strongest sections, and most likely one of yours too. Your pharmacy education has limited application for the MCAT but it is most applicable to the biology section material. Since it was my strongest baseline subject, I was able to cover the material relatively quickly and with ease.

#3: Register for the MCAT. It's important that you register early so that you can secure a spot at a local testing facility. The longer you wait the more likely you will have to travel to a distant testing center. Some applicants have to cross-state borders just to sit for the exam. There are also different sign-up time windows known as Gold, Silver, and Bronze. Each "zone" is associated with different costs with Bronze charging the most, since it is closest to the actual exam date. Essentially, the earlier you decide on an exam date, the cheaper it will be. This will also reduce the chance of having a distant test taking site. However, I would recommend that you do not sit for the exam unless you are ready. You can move your test date back if necessary and any costs you incur will pale in comparison to a terrible MCAT score.

- **Resource:** MCAT Registration
  https://students-residents.aamc.org/applying-medical-school/taking-mcat-exam/

3 MONTHS OUT:

#1: Review and learn. Any finished material should be reviewed weekly, and you should complete many practice questions along the way. Having a strong review pattern will prove useful when you begin to introduce brand new concepts from different sections.

#2: Complete practice questions/practice exams. When you finish learning new material for a particular section you should take a section bank. You may also want to time yourself to emulate test conditions. You are fighting the clock during the exam so training yourself to think quickly and efficiently will pay off. Depending on how many full-length practice exams you have at your disposal, you could also begin to take them regularly. For instance, my Princeton Review Course provided me with 10+ exams so taking an exam every 2 weeks helped me get accustomed to the MCAT format. To some, taking these exams so early may be wasteful. I had only covered biology material and some CARS content, so I performed poorly on the sections I had yet to cover. The key to this method was that it validated my study techniques when I had an excellent biology section score. Confidence is an important mental factor that cannot be overlooked.

2 MONTHS OUT:

#1: You are two months out from judgement day. Have a plan to finish all new content within a month. You will want to start taking full length CARS sections to develop your stamina. If you are particularly good at the CARS section, then this may be premature.

#2: Begin extensive review of your completed full-length exams. Analyze the questions you missed and determine the root cause of the error. Were you pressed for time and barely finished the end of the section? Were you making careless mistakes or misreading the question? Identifying these issues can help you catch yourself and avoid future errors. Not only should you review the incorrect answers but the questions you got correct as well. Did you get a question right only because of a lucky guess? There may be knowledge gaps hidden in the questions you got correct, which is a dangerous arena for future mistakes.

1 MONTH OUT:

All new content should be finished at this point, and you should enter a period of pure review along with weekly full-length MCATs. Review of each full-length should be comprehensive.

Switch over from 3rd party test prep material and utilize AAMC provided content and exams exclusively. If you want to preserve your AAMC full-lengths for the final couple weeks, then continue to utilize third-party full-lengths if necessary.

1 WEEK OUT:

Take your final 2 AAMC tests this week but make sure you give yourself at least 2 days of rest leading up to the actual exam. This should ensure you are in prime testing shape and not burnt out.

Continue your endless review and focus plenty of your effort on psychology terms. This material is the closest to pure memorization and will be best learned from cramming. The psychology section is the most similar to pharmacy style examination format so cramming this material is actually quite effective. I recommend you complete the Quizlet set below at least once a day.

- **Resource:** Psych/Soc Quizlet Deck
  https://quizlet.com/395290024/mcat-psychsociology-flash-cards/

1 DAY BEFORE:

Take a mental break, relax, and recognize that all your hard work has prepared you for this moment. Do some light review of psych/soc concepts or things you need to brush up on but do not strain yourself. Get outdoors, spend time with family, and kick back, for you are ready. Get a good night's rest and make sure you pack a good lunch with plenty of snacks for test day.

SUMMARY:

4-5 Months Out	3 Months Out	2 Months Out	1 Month Out	1 Week Left	1 Day Before
Take your 1st full-length MCAT	Start taking full-lengths bi-weekly	Continue bi-weekly full-lengths	Weekly full-lengths at a minimum	Final AAMC Tests with allotted review time	Take a mental break, relax, and do something you enjoy
Begin learning content	Continue learning content	Create a plan to finish new content within one month	Finish all new content	Extensive review with emphasis on psychology/ sociology material	
Register for the MCAT	Begin review of old content	Continue review of old material but NOT at the expense of finishing new content.	Begin an extensive review process using practice exam passages and questions		
Third Party Resources (Khan Academy, Kaplan, Princeton Review)				Switch to AAMC content exclusively	

This is a very large undertaking in and of itself, so I applaud you for trying! You are already balancing your pharmacy school responsibilities along with committing countless hours to prepare for this exam. Kudos to you! As a reminder, I am certainly not an MCAT guru, but I hope you can utilize my plan and transform it into a personal algorithm that fits you! Do your own research on different study strategies and see how they compare to this approach.

VOIDING YOUR MCAT:

At the conclusion of your official MCAT exam, you will be given the option to "void" your exam. If you decide to do so, your exam will not be scored, and all evidence of the attempt will be deleted. This option is typically reserved for students who had a disastrous test taking experience. Choosing to void may be related to some external life factors or could be as simple as having a horrible test day. Whatever the reason, you do have a final say in whether your exam should be scored.

In general, you should never void your exam based on performance issues. That is because you shouldn't sit for the exam until you are ready! With that said, you may have underestimated how prepared you really were. You may feel the need to scrap everything because you guessed on plenty of questions, ran out of time on a section, or just felt like the test was harder. I am here to tell you should control these natural emotions and avoid voiding your exam. Most students actually perform a few points higher on their actual MCAT despite these negative thoughts after test day. Also keep in mind that some students erroneously void their exam when they let their anxiety and fears control their behavior. Feeling nervous about your performance is a natural phenomenon but do not let it consume you. You probably did better than you thought! If not, a bad test score isn't the end of the world.

TAKEAWAYS:

- The MCAT is not a clinical exam and tasks applicants on a large volume of undergraduate level content.

- You can't rely on your pharmacy knowledge to get you through this exam.

- A strong MCAT score is one of the most important parts of a successful application.

- Don't skimp out on preparation material, limit your distractions, commit all your effort into this endeavor.

- AAMC provided content is as good as gold.
- Develop a study plan and stick to it.

- Push your exam back if you are falling behind or if your practice full-length scores are below your goal.

- Don't void your exam unless you absolutely have too.

PHARM.D. TO M.D.

PART FOUR:

THE PRIMARY APPLICATION

"A mind that is stretched by a new experience can never go back to its old dimensions"

– Oliver Wendell Holmes Jr.

Congrats! If you are reading this, you have likely already taken your MCAT and are looking into crafting the perfect application. As an alternative, you may just be curious to see if it gets worse than the MCAT... luckily, it does not. In this chapter we will discuss some important details concerning what you should disclose about yourself and how to do it effectively. The Primary Application is a medical school's first impression of you and your goal is to blow them away. As we know, your MCAT and GPA represent your academic competency but will do little to demonstrate who you are as a person. These statistics will keep your application out of the recycling bin, but only for so long. They get you past the bouncer at the front door, but they won't keep you in the building forever. The human component of your application is missing and is what most medical schools realistically want in the end. They still require your MCAT and GPA to be within their designated metrics, but they also recognize that a holistic and empathetic applicant will fair far better in their program. This is a tough realization that many high stat applicants face, especially when their life experiences are lackluster or when they are devoid of social capacity. So how do you tell the admissions team who you really are? You can start with drafting a rock-solid personal statement and memorable experiences for the work and activities section. You goal is to compel the admission board that you are a qualified applicant, who is dedicated to medicine and patient care. As you will see, doing this isn't always easy!

As we progress through this chapter you may have more specific questions about each individual section of the Primary Application than I am able to answer. Fortunately for you, the AAMC creates a yearly **"AMCAS Applicant Guide"** to cover every step of the process. What this guide lacks is pharmacist insight, a niche that we will explore. Feel free to reference the guide "PRN" but make sure you are utilizing the most recently updated version. This can easily be found by googling "AMCAS Applicant Guide" followed by the current year.

- **Resource:** AMCAS APPLICANT GUIDE 2021
  https://students-residents.aamc.org/media/5186/download

PRIMARY APPLICATION TIMELINE AND THE PERKS OF APPLYING EARLY:

One of the most important facets of the Primary Application is understanding the timing schedule that the application runs on. Each year the AMCAS Primary Application "Opens" in early May but cannot be formally submitted until late May or very early June. For instance, the 2021-2022 cycle had AMCAS open on May 4th, and the earliest you could submit was May 28th. **Ideally, you want to submit your application the earliest you can.** The sooner your application is in line to be "verified" the sooner medical schools will receive your application package.

When you choose to submit your primary application, the submission is permanent and very few changes can be made. There are several components that can be updated with new information including new MCAT scores. AMCAS reserves the right to address any omissions or discrepancies that may prompt further adjustment. Upon Submission, your application will be listed as "Ready for Review" and is subsequently placed in a verification queue.

Verification is the process in which AMCAS will validate your inputs and make sure your application is completely, and correctly filled out. The reasoning behind the long wait is that AMCAS employees must read your application line for line and match your course work to your transcripts. This is an extremely tedious process, so kudos to them! In order to get to the verification stage, you may have to wait several weeks; as the cycle progresses and the number of applicant submissions increases, the wait time can increase exponentially. The busiest months include June and July. According to the AAMC, during peak busy season the verification process can take up to 6 weeks, meaning your application could be sitting idle for weeks in a queue while other early applicants are already "at the baseball diamond, taking at-bats." This could result in you falling behind in the cycle and possibly hurting your chances of getting an interview invite.

An even bigger problem could include having to wait several weeks to get verified and upon inspection the reviewer finds an error in your application that cannot be adjusted without your involvement. A small mistake from a lack of careful review can delay your approval for several more weeks! Make sure you fill out your primary application with great care.

Fortunately for our procrastinators, if you don't quite submit your application on the first possible day, you won't be considered "behind schedule." Despite the opportunity to get ahead of the verification rush, AMCAS won't actually send your application to medical schools until late June. For the 2021-2022 application cycle, that date would be June 26th. You may find yourself completely verified prior to that date, but your application won't distribute to your school list until the AAMC allows it. The benefit of applying early can be seen when your application is part of the first cohort to land on each medical school's desk. This is strictly a numbers game and the sooner you can secure one of the few interview invites, the better chances you will have of getting into a program. This is the principle of rolling admissions that most medical schools employ. Let's consider a few examples to solidify this point.

PHARM.D. TO M.D.

Student A	Student B	Student C
This student submitted their primary application on the first day available. They are subsequently verified within 2 weeks. Their application will be pushed out in the first grouping to medical schools come June 26th. They receive an onslaught of secondary applications and complete them with similar haste.	This student submitted their primary in mid-June. Verification takes 4 weeks, and their application is sent to medical schools in mid-July. Secondary applications are submitted by early August.	This student submitted their primary in late July. Verification takes 6 weeks, and their application is sent to medical schools in early September. They receive secondary invites in mid-September and don't complete them until October.
Their application is as early as it gets. They have the best advantage considering their application will be among the first ones medical schools see, process, and decide to invite for interviews. This student maximized their chances by being proactive in the cycle.	They are still relatively early and will likely not incur any penalties since most interview invites have not gone out. They may be excluded from the earliest interview pool despite a quick secondary turnaround time.	This student would be considered late and has stacked the odds against themselves. It is still possible to get into a program, but a reasonable amount of their fellow applicants will have already interviewed. These interviewee veterans are far closer to securing an acceptance than poor old Student C.

    Sometimes application delays are unavoidable but do your best to stack the odds in your favor. **This is a friendly reminder to pre-write your primary application to the best of your ability.** As a pharmacy student you should dedicate the spring semester of PY3 year towards perfecting your primary application. 6 months is plenty of time to draft a personal statement and get your school list in order. Applying on-time can save you a lot of stress on the back end!

For all you PY3 MCAT retakers (including me), applying like "Student A" may not be in the cards for you. While not ideal, you can still have an extremely successful application cycle. My path resembles "Student B." I took my second MCAT after Spring PY3 finals in mid-May. I did not get my score report until mid-June and submitted my primary a few days later. After 4 weeks of waiting for verification, I was finally pushed through to the programs of my choosing. Thanks to some proactive secondary preparation, I was able to complete all my secondaries by the end of July!

As important as early application timing can be it is just one variable in this complicated process. There are additional factors that can damage your application health despite having exceptional statistics and well-to-do clinical experiences. We will address several more of these by the conclusion of this chapter.

BUILDING A STRONG APPLICATION:

As medicine evolves, medical schools have a growing interest in finding holistic candidates. We have entered an era where exceptional academic proficiency is insufficient to garner a medical school acceptance. In your research you may come across horror story posts of applicants with fabulous stats (523 MCAT and 4.0 GPA) that never got accepted, let alone a single interview. While there may have been many limitations to their application such as a late submission, a poorly crafted school list, or serial killer vibes on interview day, they were likely NOT holistic applicants. **Pure academic excellence will no longer carry an applicant through to the finish line.** Modern medicine requires students to have the ability to master conceptual data, demonstrate a devotion to service, be enthusiastic learners, and consider diversity of perspective. These are not concepts that can be learned from a textbook but are developed through experience. This is not to suggest that physicians in older generations did not demonstrate these qualities, but rather in modern medicine, these characteristics are no longer the exception but the standard. Fortunately, pharmacy students have a tremendous amount of experience so working through the primary application can be quite enjoyable. You will have the opportunity to reflect on meaningful clinical encounters that you are passionate about and will finally have the opportunity to defend your decision to leave pharmacy.

You may also be wondering, "what makes for a holistic applicant?" Check out the chart below and see for yourself.

Checklist for a Holistic Applicant:	Comments:
A Good MCAT Score:	Does your score qualify you for an Allopathic or Osteopathic track? The average accepted MD candidate had a 511.5 while the average accepted DO candidate had a 504.3.
Clinical Work Experiences Hours: (Paid and Unpaid)	<u>Unpaid Example</u>: IPPE or APPE Rotations <u>Paid Example</u>: Pharmacy Intern Position in a Hospital or Community setting
	The more hours and exposure you have the better. Clinical rotations are an excellent way to communicate with patients and effectuate a real change in their medical care. If you are practicing motivational interviewing or conducting a comprehensive medication review, you are making a difference! These are experiences that your fellow applicants will lack. Take advantage of the extra opportunities you have had and share the work you have done on your Primary Application.
Clinical and Experimental Research:	How many hours have you put forth? Did your contributions facilitate the project's advancement? If so, did you get authorship on a peer-reviewed publication or abstract? Have you presented your work via a poster at any conferences? These are all questions you must ask yourself. If you said yes to any of them, you should be in good shape.
	The general consensus is that Publications are valued the most, followed by abstracts/posters, and finally finishing with quantity of hours. For instance, you may have 1,000 hours of research experience but nothing to show for it in the form of results. While you can still reflect on the experience and formulate your endeavors into a reasonable Work/Activities submission, it will not have the same gravity as a publication. Alternatively, having several publications, doesn't mean that you get a free pass. Your reviewer or future interviewer may ask you about your work, so be prepared!
	There may be some of you reading this and having a miniature panic attack. "I don't have any research, what can I do?" I would recommend you reach out to your pharmacy school faculty to get involved in a project. Clinical projects will be much easier to carry out in a short period of time. They can also lead to multiple poster presentations from the same data source. On APPE rotations you could also work on projects, especially if you have several rotations in the same hospital system.

Physician Shadowing Hours:	I find it ironic that many applicants underestimate the significance of shadowing. How else would a student really know they belong in medicine if they have never been exposed to the line of work? Some applicants believe that their 30 hours of shadowing a family medicine physician are sufficient to authenticate a desire to become a cardiothoracic surgeon!
	As a pharmacy student making the "big switch" can be justified by racking up hundreds of shadowing hours that will validate your decision both personally and to an outside reviewer. Use these hours as leverage to compel your reviewer or interviewer that you chose this path for a reason and you can back it up with experience.
	Many traditional applicants have expressed difficulty in finding physicians to shadow. While unfortunate for them, you can take advantage of your professional relationships with physicians and ask them if you can shadow. For example, you could reach out to that doctor that always calls your pharmacy, or the physician who is running rounds in the hospital while you deliver medications. Remember it never hurts to ask and most physicians love helping those who are bold and passionate.
Conduct a Medical Mission Trip:	This experience is not absolutely necessary but is a great way to showcase what you really care about. Some applicants have even utilized their medical mission trip experiences to tie their entire application together. If you are passionate about global medicine or helping those in need, what better way to demonstrate this zeal than to prove it by crossing borders.
	One of my personal reservations with the profession of pharmacy was its lack of true patient exposure. Undertaking a medical mission trip during pharmacy school changed me forever and solidified my passion for medicine. It was on my trip that I decided that I was going to take the MCAT for the first time. A medical mission trip can be a life changing experience for you and the people you encounter along the way!

Volunteer Hours:	Admissions Committees love applicants who volunteer their time to help the community. They understand that you are ridiculously busy, especially as a pharmacy student. Therefore, dedicating your limited free time to those in need will speak volumes of your character and commitment. The hours you invest in your community will pay out 10-fold, not just in application strength, but in personal growth as well.
	While I cannot quantify the perfect number of hours needed, your aim should be in the hundreds. By the time I was applying I had only amassed approximately 70 hours and I believe it was a major drawback to my application.

Leadership Roles:	Considering the multitude of leadership opportunities in pharmacy school this should be a walk in the park. There were countless professional pharmacy organizations at my alma mater, each with their own panel of board members. These would include, ACCP, AMCP, APA, ASCP, CPNP, HERT, Kappa Epsilon, Kappa Psi, Lambda Kappa Sigma, NCPA, Phi Delta Chi, PLS, Rho Chi, PPA, PPAG, PSHP, and SNPhA. I am confident that you will be able to find a leadership role in one of these alphabet soup pharmacy organizations.
	Taking on a leadership role demonstrates responsibility and an ability to work with people. As a leader you will be tested with conflict management and challenged to collaborate with others. These are very important qualities that an admission committee looks for in its future student body.

A Strong GPA (BCPM and Non-Science)	Each medical school will have different requirements for what is considered a competitive GPA. Some programs take more interest in the sGPA while others find little value in the distinction. My only recommendation in this section is for students with a 3.0 GPA or lower to reconsider applying. Statistically speaking, applicants with such a low GPA will struggle during the cycle and will likely be filtered out even before getting a secondary application.

PHARM.D. TO M.D.

Now that we have created a template for a holistic applicant, I want to challenge you to fill it in with your own experiences. Utilize my application as an example. Also, I would like to recognize that my application was far from stellar so I encourage you to add at least 100 extra hours to each section if possible. Completing this exercise will help you plan the "Work and Activities" section on your Primary Application. Brainstorming with this template can help organize what you want to talk about and dig-up past experiences you may have forgotten!

NATHAN M. GARTLAND

Checklist for a Holistic Applicant:	My Application:	Your Application:
A Good MCAT Score:	First Attempt 497 (38th Percentile)	
	Second Attempt 510 (80th Percentile)	
Clinical Work Experiences Hours: (Paid and Unpaid)	1st APPE Rotation – 210 Unpaid hours	
	Hospital Pharmacy Intern – 1,000 Paid hours	
Clinical and Experimental Research:	Experimental Cancer Project – 540 hours	
	Experimental Pain Project – 70 hours (One Publication)	
	Clinical Research – 200 hours	
Physician Shadowing Hours:	Dr. "X" – 25 hours	
	Dr. "Y" – 30 hours	
	Dr. "Z" – 72 hours	
Conduct a Medical Mission Trip:	Cap-Haitien, Haiti – 80 hours	
Volunteer Hours:	Event "A" – 25 hours	
	Event "B" – 50 hours	
	Event "C" – 120 hours	
Leadership Roles:	President of Phi Delta Chi – 600 hours	
	Phi Lambda Sigma Board – 40 hours	
A Strong GPA (BCPM and Non-Science)	Cumulative GPA – 3.78	
	Science (BCPM) GPA – 3.91	
Final Results:	28 MD Programs (AMCAS), and 6 DO Programs (AACOMAS)	
	Approximately 28 Secondaries	
	4 MD and 3 DO Interview Invites	
	1 MD acceptance and withdrawal from all other programs	

THE PRIMARY APPLICATION LAYOUT:

We will now discuss the various sections of the AMCAS Primary Application. Since you are now well equipped to fill out each component, we can begin to work through the application piece by piece. Remember, if you get lost or confused you can always refer back to the **AMCAS Applicant Guide** to clarify. Additionally, if you haven't made an AAMC account yet you will need to do so to proceed to the AMCAS Sign in page.

INITIAL STEPS:

Your first prompt should involve verification of your AAMC information associated with your account. This will be followed with a variety of personal questions related to your birth, sex, schools attended, degrees obtained, etc. Complete these questions and continue to the "Transcripts Section." This can be a tedious and confusing portion of the AMCAS application. It is also a common reason that applications get delayed. Make sure you order transcripts utilizing the custom AMCAS Pre-Barcoded Transcript Request Form assigned to your application. Contact your university registrar to make sure they can send an official PDF eTranscript to AMCAS on your behalf. This process is time consuming and can be rather frustrating, especially if you have to coordinate with your registrar. If you are ordering official transcripts at this point you will also want to order an official copy for yourself. You will need it in the Coursework section of the application, so might as well "kill two birds with one stone."

INSTITUTIONAL ACTION:

If you have a history of any institutional action (IA) regarding unacceptable academic performance or conduct violation you are obligated to answer "yes" in this portion of the application. You are also expected to answer "yes" even if your action has been deleted or expunged from your official transcripts. Failure to truthfully do so can result in an investigation of your application.

This portion of the application can make any applicant nervous, even those who have a polished record. **For the students with a small blemish or two, I want to reassure you that it is not the end of the world.** Having to disclose an IA is not ideal but it will not stop you from getting into medical school. With that said, the severity of the infraction and the quantity of violations will count against you. For instance, a conduct violation from freshmen year will fair far better than an academic integrity violation within the last 6 months. The further back the infraction is the better off you will be and in general, behavioral infractions are less severe than academic integrity breaches. Being the morally onerous pharmacy student that you are, I don't anticipate any IA's being a problem for you. Alas if you do have a blemish in your past, you should read the Student Doctor Network article below about taking potential legal action to protect your application chances.

There is without a doubt a stigma against institutional actions and unfortunately the consequences of disclosing one can have real life implications for your application. It is impossible to quantify how the odds are stacked against an IA disclosing applicant but many still get accepted every year. Fortunately, I was one of them. An important step to handling an IA is to own up to your mistake and recognize that you could have acted differently. You must accept the consequences for your actions and utilize the experience as momentum to facilitate personal and professional growth.

Lastly, if you answer "yes" to having an IA, I promise you it will NOT be the last time you are asked about it. It will come up at plenty of interviews and some institutions will request a formal report form your university's office of student conduct. Hint hint, don't lie on the AMCAS about what happened!

- **Resource:** Student Doctor Network IA Support
  https://www.studentdoctor.net/2020/02/13/legal-matters-institutional-action-basics/

COURSEWORK:

If you are reading this and are actually preparing to submit your AMCAS within the next 1-2 months, stop what you are doing and go to your university's registrar website to order your official transcripts. You will want an official copy so that you can input every course you have ever taken at said university. If you took courses at a different school for undergrad or took my elective credit advice you will also need transcripts from that institution. Even if you transferred the credits into your pharmacy school, AMCAS requires a transcript from the original course providing institution. Do not use an unofficial transcript as some information may be different.

As you input the course information into the application you will have to classify the courses starting with Academic Year and Term. According to AMCAS, a "year" starts in the summer and ends with the spring. This is an important distinction. For instance, at my pharmacy school I was required to complete my IPPE I and II rotations over the summer. I completed my IPPE I course in the summer of 2017. Although my university considered this course as part of the 2016-2017 academic year, AMCAS would consider it 2017-2018. Keep this in mind if you have taken any summer courses.

You will then be asked to designate a "year in school" for each course. This is an important classification because AMCAS will calculate a specific GPA for each year of school. The options include High School, Freshman, Sophomore, Junior, Senior, Postbaccalaureate, and Graduate. Your pharmacy level courses will fall in the Graduate (GR) designation. If for some reason that is not an available option, you can designate your content as Senior (SR).

Now comes the tedious part. You will need to input the exact course number and name into the application. It is imperative that you do this correctly or there will be delays in your verification processing. The laborious nature of this individual step can rival the annoyance of studying for the MCAT. You have been warned!

Upon thoroughly inputting the course information you are now ready for the Course Classification assignment. While inappropriately classifying a course may not hold up the processing of your application, **AMCAS does reserve the right to change any designation you assigned**, especially if they believe it is incorrectly labeled or a different classification is more appropriate. This portion is critical for applicants because the **final classification will be used to calculate your BCPM GPA (sGPA) and your AO GPA (all other courses).** You already know your total GPA from your official transcript but have likely not calculated your BCPM GPA yet. You can do so at Medical School Headquarters using their online GPA calculator. This is not an exercise you will want to pass up on. AMCAS will NOT calculate any of your GPA's until you have officially submitted your application and have been verified by a reviewer. Having your courses inputted in this calculator can also show you how your sGPA will change based on how you designate different courses. Remember that sGPA is important because "science" related courses are often considered more challenging. Having a high sGPA demonstrates academic excellence in difficult courses and medical school admissions committees recognize this.

- **Resource:** Medical School HQ GPA Calculator
  https://medicalschoolhq.net/med-school-gpa-calculator-for-amcas-aacomas-and-tmdsas/

So how do you classify a course? According to the AMCAS Applicant Guide, **Course classifications are based on the primary content of the course.** It's that simple and to be honest rather lenient. As a pharmacy student the courses you take are uncommon in the eyes of most reviewers and therefore it affords you some degree of flexibility in how you classify pharmacy content. A list of possible classifications you can choose from includes Biology (BIOL), Chemistry (CHEM), Physics (PHYS), Mathematics (MATH), Business (BUSI), Communications (COMM), Computer Science and Technology (COMP), Behavioral and Social Sciences (BESS), Education (EDUC), Engineering (ENGI), English Language and Literature (ENGL), Fine Arts (ARTS), Foreign Languages Linguistics and Literature (FLAN), Government Law and Political Science (GOVT), Health Sciences (HEAL), History (HIST), Natural and Physical Sciences (NPSC), Philosophy and Religion (PHIL), and Other (OTHR). A rather exhaustive list that only scratches the surface.

These topics can be further broken down into subcategories that will help you sort your coursework more efficiently. I recommend you look at the comprehensive chart found on page 36 of the **AMCAS Applicant Guide** for more information. For Convenience you can also check out the individual chart.

- **Resource:** AMCAS® Course Classification Guide
  https://students-residents.aamc.org/media/7861/download

You should be familiar with the Health Sciences (HEAL) classification because you will utilize it frequently. Under this umbrella term is the "Pharmacology and Pharmacy" subclassification. You'll also notice that this terminology is extremely vague and provides little assistance in classifying the variety of pharmacy classes you have taken. Unfortunately, if you classify a course under HEAL it will not count towards your sGPA.

This can be rather frustrating when some of the most challenging and clinically oriented courses in pharmacy are excluded from the sGPA. This is especially true if you excelled in these classes! While it may not be the case for everyone, I found myself performing far better in clinical pharmacy classes than I ever did in undergraduate physics or chemistry. Based off this metric, that "B-" in general physics is more valuable than your "A+" in Therapeutics of the Critically Ill. As you know pharmacy level courses are far more difficult than the majority of undergraduate level classes so your GPA may be artificially lower than other applicants. A traditional pre-health applicant with a 3.6 sGPA would be considered equivalent to a Pharmacy Students sGPA of 3.6 despite having graduate level workload. Unfortunately, you are competing against some of these inflated GPAs when the course load many undergraduates have completed is nowhere near the same level of difficulty as a pharmacy school semester. It is a reality that many pharmacy students must come to terms with.

Classification is rather simple until you reach the professional years of your schooling. In undergrad the courses fit the description that AMCAS puts forth far better than most pharmacy related content. For example, an undergraduate level Biology class would be classified as BIOL and a history class would fall under HIST. Great, but how would you classify Pharmacy Law and Ethics? Would it fall under "Government (GOVT)" or "Health Sciences (HEAL)." In general, this level of minutiae is inconsequential, and you'll notice that both Government and Health sciences are excluded from the sGPA calculation, so it doesn't really matter.

Let's try another example. You will likely have taken Infectious Disease I and II as part of your pharmacy curriculum. Would this fall under "Health Sciences (HEAL)" and be excluded from your sGPA or "Biology (BIOL)" under the microbiology subclassification? You are now left to discern where this falls and picking can introduce a whole new stressor to the application cycle. This is also an opportunity to consider how the classification would impact your sGPA. If you received an "A+," it would be in your best interest to classify it as BIOL so that the credits are used to bolster your sGPA. If you received a "C+," it may be in your best interest to label it as HEAL and the credits would be excluded from your sGPA.

Focusing on a single class will hardly influence your sGPA but making this adjustment for every class in pharmacy school can lead to a high sGPA calculation. In the end it doesn't change your overall GPA but you can classify things to fit your interests!

As a disclaimer, I am NOT suggesting that you mislabel courses. You are still obligated to classify them based on the primary content of the course according to AMCAS. In the end you are still responsible for the integrity of your designations. You also cannot make this adjustment to courses that are clearly mislabeled. For instance, your "A+" in your undergraduate writing course would never fall under BIOL. If you designate it so, your reviewer will make the correction. My recommendation is to take advantage of the ambiguity of pharmacy level course classifications to benefit your sGPA calculation, just do so truthfully!

TAKEAWAYS:

- Order a copy of your official transcripts from your university's registrar.

- AMCAS will not conduct any GPA calculations until after you have submitted your primary application.

- Your course classifications are used to calculate sGPA and other GPA.

- AMCAS reserves the right to change any classification if they deem it necessary.

- Your sGPA is more valuable than your total GPA or any other calculated GPA through AMCAS.

WORK/ACTIVITIES SECTION:

In this section you will have the opportunity to write about up to 15 experiences and highlight the uniqueness of your application. This could include a work experience, participation in extracurriculars, honors, awards, research projects, shadowing experiences, medical mission trips, a meaningful patient interaction, or anything else that you believe will broadcast who you are. For example, I wrote about my passion for learning to play the piano from watching YouTube© videos. You will also have the opportunity to declare up to 3 of the experiences as "most meaningful." As a reminder, ordinary activity descriptions are limited to 700 characters while most meaningful are awarded up to 1,325 characters. These extra characters should be used to clarify why this experience was so important to you.

If you have been following my schedule, you will have likely pre-written the experience descriptions and you will be able to input them with relative ease. During the input process you will have to fill out additional information about the experience. This includes designating the experience type, experience name, experience dates, total hours, organization name if affiliated, country/city of occurrence, contact information of a supervisor, and the pre-written description.

You may also be wondering, "In what order will my experiences appear on my application?" The order in which you create and add your experiences will be the permanent order regarding AMCAS but are subject to rearrangement by medical schools. The reason being that most medical schools prefer to rearrange the experiences to highlight categories that interest them (shadowing, research etc.). This is a non-factor, so input the experiences in the order that best suits you!

PHARM.D. TO M.D.

HOW TO WRITE
A WORK/ACTIVITIES DESCRIPTION:

Before you can even start you should create a bulleted list of experiences to serve as an outline. Throughout pharmacy school I had kept a Google-document with descriptions of every important event that I felt would benefit a resume. I would recommend you do the same. Even if you don't use it here, it will save you plenty of time when drafting a Curriculum Vitae (CV), a necessary document for professional pharmacists. My document served as an excellent template to help me easily create a running list of experiences. I have provided this list below as an example. My most meaningful experiences are designated with "**MM**" lettering.

1. Other – 1st APPE Rotation in a Hospital

2. Physician Shadowing resulting in clinical intervention (**MM**)

3. Physician Shadowing

4. Clinical Research Experience – Retrospective Chart Review (**MM**)

5. Community Service Outreach Event – Medically Related

6. Pharmacy Intern Employment at a Major Hospital

7. Leadership Experience – President of a Professional Pharmacy Fraternity

8. Medical Mission Trip to Haiti (**MM**)

9. Community Service Outreach Volunteer – Non-Medically Related

10. Research Publication – Experimental Research Project

11. Leadership Experience – Phi Lambda Sigma (PLS)

12. Community Service Outreach Event – Medically Related

13. Research Program – Experimental Research Project

14. Political Advocacy – Advocate for Broaden Access to Healthcare

15. Hobbies – Amateur Piano Player

Your goal should be to portray yourself and your mission to the admissions board. Each experience should reveal a small amount of information about what you are passionate about while your personal statement ties all of these pieces together into one story. It's also fine, and recommended by some, to incorporate the same experience you list in the work/activities section into your personal statement. The cache is that you should attempt to describe the experience from a different angle or highlight a different aspect that was beneficial to you or others.

Also, when choosing which experiences to include, remember that admissions committees love holistic applicants. If you love research, certainly share your contributions but don't write-up 7 experiences just about research. You want to find the perfect balance of sharing as much as you can about yourself while avoiding lack-luster descriptions of events. Demonstrate that you are a well-rounded applicant with multiple strengths.

So how do you write an accurate, insightful, yet purposeful description of an experience? According to Shemmassian Academic Consulting, you should utilize the outline listed below. After you have filled in the template you should be able to easily construct a paragraph style description that is concise yet compelling.

- Time Spent:

- Responsibilities/Accomplishments:

- Impact on You or People Involved:

- Qualities Demonstrated:

- Lessons Learned or Personal Growth from this Experience:

EXTERNAL RESOURCES:

- **Resource: 2021 AMCAS Work/Activities**
  https://www.shemmassianconsulting.com/blog/amcas-work-and-activities#amcas-work-and-activities-categories

MOST MEANINGFUL EXPERIENCES:

When it comes to there are several minor tips to discuss regarding how to designate them and how to write them. You may still utilize the ordinary experience template if you see fit. One caveat of designating an experience as most meaningful is that you are given a higher character limit, indicating that you should portray insightful reflection. Consider this the intermediary between a personal statement and an ordinary experience description. Courtesy of **Cracking Med School Admissions,** here are 5 tips that will improve your most meaningful experience reflections.

- **Tell a Story** – This is an abstract, not a novel. It is also a way to highlight a unique experience or story that you may not want to share in your personal statement.

- **Differentiate Yourself** – Everyone will have had patient experiences, but hardly any will have had the same involvement as a pharmacy student. Use this to your advantage and talk about the connection you made, not just the outcomes.

- **Maintain your Mission and Overall Narrative** – For instance, if you love cancer research and have made that apparent, talking about a cancer patient you encountered will reinforce that narrative.

- **Emphasize the Impact** – If your involvement resulted in a subjective or objective benefit, share these specific details to add value to your description. For example, if you have participated in a COVID-19 Vaccination Clinic, share the number of shots you provided or the number of people you triaged to combat the pandemic.

- **Connect to the Future** – If an experience was meaningful to you in the past, how has it better prepared you for the future? Has this experience broadened your perspective, and will it make you a better physician in the end? These are the kinds of introspective questions the admissions committee loves to see answered on an application.

MISCHELLANTEOUS TIPS:

#1: Proofread everything at least 10 times and over a 3-day period. You will be amazed at how many typos you will find or awkwardly worded sentences you will catch. The last thing you want are careless typos detracting from the amazing experiences you are sharing. A lazy submission can hurt your credibility as a healthcare professional.

#2: You can't write about APPEs unless you have completed the experience or are currently participating in one at the time of submission. I picked a majority of my APPE rotations under the guise that I would be able to boast the complexity and prestige of the program on my Work/Activities section. As you know this was far from the truth and quite naive on my end. How can you write about the impact an experience has had on you if you haven't even started the experience? I was tempted to write about my future hematological malignancy rotation at Johns Hopkins but was forced to leave it off the application.

#3: Hour verification fact or fiction? You may be wondering, "Does AMCAS verify hours and experiences with your listed reference?" While you are still inclined to accurately and honestly present information on your application, the truth is that they generally DO NOT verify. Most medical schools receive over 10,000 applications. They hardly have time to send you an email correspondence about your application status let alone contact each and every reference on a students work/activities section. Assuming that of those 10,000 students each one on average submits 10 experiences, one medical school would have to follow-up with 100,000 inquiries. Unrealistic and quite frankly a waste of time, especially to verify that "Jimmy completed 35 volunteer hours at the homeless shelter and not the 45 he reported." Please don't use this as a reason to bolster your hours. Just because it's unlikely to get caught doesn't mean you won't. I certainly wouldn't want to be the applicant that gets investigated.

#4: You don't have to submit all 15 experiences in the work/activities section. You can do as little as you choose. If you can only conjure up 11 experiences, then so be it. Although, I would recommend you attempt to complete all 15 if possible. The more information you can provide to bolster your application the better chances you have at securing an interview slot. With that said, if you are clearly out of content to write or reflect upon, please don't fill in the extra slots with meaningless examples. The lack of quality will feel out of place compared to the rest of your experiences and may even subtract from your overall application narrative.

LETTERS OF RECOMMENDATION:

Letters of Evaluation are essential to a holistic medical school application. Medical schools understand that you will do everything in your power to craft your application to fit the ideal applicant model, regardless of how realistic it is. Because of this reality, you are encouraged to get several letters of evaluation to serve as your external spokesperson. The status of your letter writer and quality of the content can help validate the information you have already provided, while adding more about your persona and character as an individual. Most medical schools require 2-3 letters of recommendation while others require a minimum of 5. I would recommend you have at least 5 letters to be safe. You can submit a maximum of 10 letters into the AMCAS application, but this quantity of letters is far above the average and honestly, quite unnecessary. Remember, when it comes to letter evaluations, quality over quantity.

Additionally, letters of recommendation are the only portion of the Primary Application that you can add after a submission besides a new MCAT score. This is important because you are able to maintain your submission deadline and stay on schedule despite having a missing letter. AMCAS works with applicants because they don't want a lazy letter writer to hold up a student's medical school application, at least initially.

LETTER SUBTYPES:

There are different types of letters of evaluation that you can submit. This would include a Committee Letter (CL), a Letter Package (LP), and an Individual Letter (IL). A CL holds the most weight when considering the letter hierarchy. This is because a CL includes your university's personalized evaluation of you along with, or without, a packaged file of your additional letters of recommendation. Not only do you have 5-6 letter writers approving of you individually, but you have the backing of your institution's pre-health committee. Unfortunately, unless you have been in contact with your university's pre-health committee and are enrolled in a formal pre-health program, **you will NOT have access to a CL.** This can be a frustrating process as some medical schools require a CL or will ask why it was not included. This is often a salvageable setback and can be remedied by communicating with the institution's admissions office. In my experience, I had to follow-up with 2 medical schools who left my application status "incomplete" for several weeks while I coordinated with the admissions clerkship.

An LP is a package of your individual letters of recommendation put together by your institution but outside the pre-health department. This also excludes the universities personalized blessing which separates it from a CL. If you are unable to formally get involved in a pre-health program or get access to a CL, an LP may be a practical way to submit your recommendations. You can contact your university's career center for further details.

An IL is rather self-explanatory and is simply a single letter of recommendation. I was unaware of the different ways to package a letter at the time of my AMCAS submission date, so I utilized 5 ILs in my Primary Application. Additionally, without the support or guidance from an institutional advisory board I had to upload these sealed documents to AMCAS through a 3rd party letter service company.

HOW TO REQUEST A LETTER OF RECOMMENDATION:

As a pharmacy student you will have likely had far more interaction with your graduate school's faculty. Pharmacy class sizes are smaller, and a majority of faculty professors are very involved in pharmacy organizations or mentoring. Your access to highly qualified letter writers is far better than most traditional pre-health applicants, who must fight tooth and nail to get an undergraduate professor to acknowledge their existence. You will have ample opportunities throughout pharmacy school to work with your professors in a variety of ways including professional organizations, regular course curriculum, preceptorship on rotations, or research, just to name a few. Your pharmacy school may also provide pharmacy students with a faculty mentor to usher them through the 4-year graduate degree. I can't think of a better letter writing candidate than a personal mentor whom you have come to know over years of growth and knowledge expansion. These examples above are also only pulling on your professional academic relationships. You may be an intern at a large hospital pharmacy or retail setting that has many supervisors whom I am sure would love to write a letter for you. Letters from family members, clergy, "family friends," or those who haven't worked directly with you in a professional setting will be regarded as weak letters of recommendation. Even if the content is positively glowing, the biased relationship can hurt the credibility of the letter. I recommend you avoid asking members of this cohort unless you have some extenuating circumstances.

Now that you have identified potential letter writers through your academic endeavors or extracurricular involvement, you need to estimate the letter quality of your potential candidates. Your best bet is to request a letter with someone whom you have worked with extensively or have a shared experience that they can relate to you. Particularly one that has demonstrated your character as a person, your compassion for others, or strong work ethic. What I mean is that you want your letter writer to be your research mentor and not the floater pharmacist you see once every two months. You should seek out faculty that you have established a deep professional connection with or your boss who has worked with you since you were a technician. My point is that exceptional letters come from exceptional relationships and these quality experiences make a letter of recommendation glow. This is an important feature when the primary goal is to stand out against the backdrop of thousands of other qualified applicants.

So how do you ask? Hopefully, you will have been hinting at pursuing a career in medicine especially leading up to the request. You want your potential letter writer to understand that this is something you are passionate about and you don't want to blindside them with the news. Your request should be in-person if possible. This is a professional courtesy that demonstrates respect and maturity on your end. **When asking, it is imperative that you formally ask for a "POSITIVE or STRONG" Letter of Recommendation.** It may seem crazy to make this distinction, but I have heard horror stories of letter writers sinking applications because of unprofessional requests or simply asking a distant writer. By asking for a basic letter of recommendation you may also end up with a weakly drafted letter that comes across as generic and unauthentic. An almost equally damaging result in the eyes of an admission's committee. Following the old English idiom, your application may be "dammed by faint praise." Requesting a "positive or strong" letter can emphasize the importance of your request and help avoid mediocre, and dare I say negative letter writing.

After your letter writer has confirmed their willingness to write you a letter, you will need to draft a follow-up email discussing several important points. You will need to comment on Letter Submission Deadlines, Letter Delivery Services Utilized, and Attach a Letter Writing Guide designed by AAMC. As mentioned in the schedule section, you will want to have your letter writers confirmed by the spring semester of your PY3 year. This should give your writers plenty of time to craft a quality letter. With regards to submission deadlines, I recommend you request that your letter be complete by mid-March and late-April at the latest. This will grant you plenty of reserve time for any unintended delays. Regarding your delivery service, you will need to mention either "Interfolio" or the "AMCAS Letter Writer Application." We will discuss which letter service is best for you in the next subsection including upload details and confidentiality agreements.

Lastly, you will want to attach a guide put forth by AAMC to help your letter writer with crafting a quality work. Writing a medical school letter of recommendation is no easy task and asking someone who may have never written one can be overwhelming. Make this process as seamless and straight forward as possible for them! **In summary, your follow-up email should include transparent deadlines, letter delivery method description, and the attached letter writing guide.** Although not always necessary, providing them with your Curriculum Vitae (CV) can also have merit.

- **Resource:** AAMC Letter Writing Guidelines
  https://www.aamc.org/system/files?file=2019-09/lettersguidelinesbrochure.pdf

As a final recommendation, you should attempt to get letter writers whom you have interacted with across a variety of experiences. This recommendation does not overrule the quality requirement. For example, you would fare better if you had 1 quality letter from an employer, a faculty member, and a community outreach supervisor instead of just 3 quality letters from the same employer. The variety of letter sources adds strength to your application. You want each letter to provide supporting evidence to the glamorous application you have already crafted. **Lastly, one of your letter writers should be a physician.** As an individual who has already forgone a career in medicine, a letter of commendation from them will hold significant weight. If you are planning on applying to osteopathic medical schools, you may also need a letter from a licensed osteopathic physician. While not absolutely necessary to apply in general, some programs will reject you outright if you do not provide them with an osteopathic letter of recommendation. This happened to me!

LETTER DELIVERY METHODS:

There are two primary letter delivery methods available to you. This would include the "AMCAS Letter Writer Application" and "Interfolio." In general, if you have a committee letter (CL) or letter package (LP) from your institution, you will likely be instructed to utilize the AMCAS Letter Writer Application. Considering a pre-health advisor must be involved to some degree to even get a CL, you should follow their individualized instruction. Interfolio is often reserved for students who plan to submit individual letters (IL) and/or will be submitting letters to both Allopathic (AMCAS) and Osteopathic (AACOMAS) application platforms. Considering most pharmacy students will fall under the Interfolio category, I will focus on this delivery method. I personally utilized Interfolio during my application cycle and found their service to be accommodating and easy to work with.

INTERFIOLIO:

#1: To begin you will want to create a **Dossier Deliver Account** through Interfolio. The cost of the service is $48. You may be tempted to sign-up for the free version, but it will NOT allow you to deliver your letters of recommendation into AMCAS or AACOMAS. You will have to upgrade to the paid service eventually, no getting around it!

#2: From the home page, on the dropdown menu select "Letters." On the top right side of the page will be a rectangle with the words "Request a Letter." Select this option and fill out the prompts. You will want to have already confirmed your letter writers prior to proceeding. After completing the online prompt, your writer will receive a communication from Interfolio with letter submission details. It is important that you inform your letter writer that this Interfolio email will be coming.

#3: Ensure that the confidentiality box <u>remains</u> checked. If it is not, your letter of recommendation will be completely worthless. Medical school admission committees expect that you will not have access to written letters and any breach of this will invalidate the letters credibility and possibly your own.

#4: When communicating with your letter writer, you should request that they produce your letter on "Professional Letter Head." Part of Interfolio's service is to not only confidentially protect letters but to determine the authenticity of the letter. Each letter will be subject to a **quality check**, which can be a useful mechanism to protect the integrity of your application. Your letters are being sent to medical schools and unprofessionally drafted letters can hurt your application. For instance, you may have the best letter writer on the planet but if they submit a poorly formatted word document with plain text, they are undermining the professionalism of letter. Interfolio will verify to see if the following details are found on your letter.

- A signature is present

- There is official letterhead

- Ensures that the writer properly uploaded a letter and not an incorrect document

- The letter had your name and the letter writer's name

- Confirm that the letter is legible

While this may seem like extra work on your end, it's really a failsafe for you to protect your letter submissions. My only qualm during this process was that I didn't know about the quality checks and had to badger my letter writers to make adjustments to the work they had already submitted. **When you reach out to your letter writers make sure you are clear-cut with what you want in each letter and what Interfolio demands to pass the quality check.**

#5: Submit your New Letter Request.

#6: Once your letter writer has finished their end of the bargain, you will need to deliver your letter to AMCAS or AACOMAS. This process is relatively straight forward so I will have you refer to Interfolio's delivery instructions. Along with these instructions includes a short 3 minute video covering each step. Check out the delivery instructions online for guidance. You will also want to check out page 54 of the **AMCAS Applicant Guide** for creating a letter entry.

#7: Once your letters of recommendation are inputted into your application portal (AMCAS/AACOMAS), you will need to assign them to each specific medical school. We will discuss this further in the Medical Schools section. I only bring it up because you will have the opportunity to choose which letters are sent to each school. For example, not everyone is able to get a total of 5 letters, let alone quality ones. You may have had to ask a person you are not too familiar with or have limited connections with. Perhaps they even told you that they wouldn't be able to craft a strong letter, but you needed the extra content. Remember, some medical schools require up to 5 letters of recommendation to be eligible for consideration. If you want to avoid having this particularly weak letter from being sent to every program on your list, you can pick and choose where it goes. This is only for students utilizing ILs. CLs and LPs are packaged and processed as a unit. AMCAS does not divide them up for distribution purposes.

TAKEAWAYS:

- Get quality, positive, strong letters of recommendation.

- Get a physician letter and specifically an osteopathic physician if you are planning on applying to osteopathic programs.

- Ask for a letter of recommendation early and in person.

- Be transparent about deadlines, disclose delivery service requirements, provide a letter writing guide, and your personal CV when contacting your letter writers.

- Interfolio is the preferred letter delivery service for most pharmacy applicants.

EXTERNAL RESOURCES:

- **Resource:** Interfolio Dossier Login
  https://www.interfolio.com/products/dossier/?gclid=Cj0KC
  Qjw9O6HBhCrARIsADx5qCQVVmf5qS41stWH8qsowm
  ucrx3zhCsgMbDCzEtYEBaUusHB8MUY41caAsNCEAL
  w_wcB

- **Resource:** Interfolio Quality Checks
  https://www.interfolio.com/resources/blog/quality-check-on-letters/

- **Resource:** Interfolio Delivery Instructions
  https://support.interfolio.com/m/62586/l/646844-how-to-use-dossier-deliver-for-a-medical-or-dental-school-application

MEDICAL SCHOOLS:

Welcome to one of the most exciting parts of the Primary Application! You are finally ready to craft your medical school list. Although the idea of picking a few schools may seem simplistic, this process has several pitfalls that can completely derail even the most successful applications. **A smart school list can be just as important as getting a quality MCAT score.** We will focus on avoiding these mistakes and help you build a comprehensive medical school list.

Before starting with this section, you will need to purchase the Medical School Admission Requirements platform, also known as the **MSAR**. The total cost for a 1-year subscription is $28 and, in my opinion, the best money you will spend during the application cycle, besides an acceptance deposit! Through the MSAR you will have access to every allopathic medical school's statistics. This includes average accepted GPAs, MCAT scores, demographics, in-state/out-of-state preferences, and far more. You will 100% need this to build a solid and informative medical school application list. We will start by addressing principles of choosing medical schools and end with how to process them in your AMCAS application.

- **Resource:** MSAR Login
  https://students-residents.aamc.org/medical-school-admission-requirements/medical-school-admission-requirements-applicants

PRINCIPLES OF PICKING MEDICAL SCHOOLS

There are a variety of important considerations to take note of when creating your school list. These include tuition cost, in-state/out-of-state bias, school mission, location, low-yield programs, average GPA, and average MCAT. While these concepts may seem intuitive, you must understand that any shortcoming can send your application to the bottom of the pile. Let us review a few basic principles that you should be familiar with as we progress through this subsection.

Important Terminology:	
Top-20 (T-20):	Medical School ranking list put forth by U.S. News every year evaluating programs based on research and primary care.
Low-Yield Programs (LYPs):	Medical schools with over 10,000 applicants per application cycle or those with abnormally small class sizes (< 60 students).
Legacy Advantage:	This is a particular advantage that is granted to applicants who are applying to a medical school in which a parent or relative graduated from. The idea being that "we liked your mother, so we will probably like you." The weight of a legacy is dependent on the specific school of interest. Some programs do not consider legacy at all.

Yield Protection:	This is the idea that an admissions committee at an institution will reject or wait-list highly qualified applicants on the grounds that such students are going to be accepted at more prestigious programs. In other words, they don't want to waste time offering an applicant a seat when they will likely jump ship when a better offer comes along. For instance, an applicant with a 523 MCAT, 4.0 GPA, and Nobel Prize worthy extracurriculars is not going to end up at a mid-tier medical school. The mid-tier program recognizes that this applicant is T-20 worthy and will paradoxically reject said student.
Rolling Admissions:	A practice for medical schools to invite students for interviews and accept them on a rolling basis. The earlier you submit, the fewer people you'll be completing against for spots. Alternatively, the later you submit your application, the greater the competition for fewer spots.

ORGANIZING YOUR SCHOOL LIST:

When creating a list of medical schools, you will need to subdivide these schools into 3 categories. The first grouping is for your "Safety schools," The second grouping is for your "Target schools", and the third grouping is for your "Reach schools." As you look through the MSAR data you will want to first look at the average MCAT and GPA. Pay close attention to each institution MCAT score as this is how you will filter programs. My personal rule of thumb is to take your own MCAT score and add 3-4 points or subtract 3-4 points. By doing so you will have created a synthetic range of MCAT scores that will represent which programs you have a realistic opportunity at getting into. For example, I got a 510 on my MCAT so my school range was 506-514. You can also look at the MSAR and see each school MCAT distribution. A reach program can be defined as a school where your MCAT falls below the 25th percentile while a safety is when your score is above the 75th percentile. To keep track of this data I created a google spreadsheet and listed each school's name underneath the appropriate grouping based on their average MCAT score. I recommend you do the same as this is only the first step to organizing the data. Each school that you list will need to be individually vetted to ensure that you have a realistic chance of getting in. I have provided a table below demonstrating this process for you to view. The MSAR may also provide you with a similar organizing tool, but I found my own methods to be just as effective and more customizable.

Safety Schools			Target Schools			Reach Schools		
506	507	508	509	510	511	512	513	514

There is no exact science to this process so please don't neglect programs entirely outside of each respective zone. If you have a compelling reason to apply to extreme reach programs, do it! Some of these reasons include the medical school is part of your undergraduate college/pharmacy school, the program is one of your state-schools, you have a legacy advantage, or have an influential letter writer with substantial academic or political pull.

IN-STATE/OUT-OF-STATE BIAS:

Now that you have organized each medical school to fit into your safety, target, and reach template you can begin investigating each program with greater scrutiny. One easy way to immediately narrow down the size of your list is to look at an individual school's in-state/out-of-state bias. This can be found by looking in the matriculated/accepted student demographics. Programs that have hardly any out-of-state students demonstrate a bias against these applicants. For example, Florida State University has a 0.1% out-of-state acceptance rate compared to a 5.3% in-state acceptance rate. Another example is Marshal University in West Virginia which has a 0.8% out-of-state acceptance rate compared to 45.5% in-state acceptance rate. Despite these schools having relatively low MCAT scores compared to other programs, you may have been tempted to group these institutions under your "safety school" category. This can be deceptive considering you realistically have little to no chance of getting in if you are an out-of-state applicant.

Your counter argument may be that "some out-of-state students make it in every year, so why won't it be me?" A reasonable suggestion, but in all likelihood, those out-of-staters had family connections to the area, grew up in the region, attended the medical school's undergraduate program, or completed a post-baccalaureate at the medical school itself. These applicants can make a convincing argument on interview day that most out-of-staters cannot. Like most medical schools, these programs want to encourage their graduated physicians to remain local and build up the healthcare system. They are looking for out-of-state applicants with ties to the area that will keep them rooted! Also keep in mind that not every medical school has an in-state/out-of-state bias. There are plenty of programs that will disregard this distinction. The unfortunate reality is that most of these programs are top-20 programs (T-20) and/or low-yield schools. We will discuss low-yield programs in a little bit.

PHARM.D. TO M.D.

Let's run through a quick example to hammer home these important points. Let's say you are from Kansas and are researching a school in Florida. You have no ties to the area and have no family within 1,000 miles of this school's location. You don't have a legacy advantage or any particularly powerful letter writers. You check the MSAR and find that this Florida school received 5,000 applications last cycle. Of those 5,000 they interviewed 10 out-of-state applicants, but only accepted 1. Would this be a smart school to apply too? Of course not! Even if your MCAT is 10 points higher than the school average you are fighting a losing battle. Pay attention to the numbers because it will save you a lot of money and time. In the end, you will have to make these decisions for yourself. You'll have to discern if the extra $200 cost per school is worth the 0.8% chance of securing an acceptance.

Now that you are aware of the impact your home-state status can have on medical school acceptances, it's time that we change the perspective. While you may be disadvantaged to apply to programs that would consider you out-of-state, the counterbalance is preferential treatment in your home-state. If you were from West-Virginia or Florida, then the previous examples were probably the most encouraging thing you have read from this book! The same holds true for other state-schools although there are exceptions like I mentioned. **The golden rule to applying to medical schools is to apply to EVERY program within your home-state.** Statistically speaking you have the best odds of getting into these programs simply because of your residence. With that said, you should also be realistic about your GPA and MCAT statistics. For example, I am from New York State and there are approximately 15 allopathic medical schools in this state alone. This large pool of schools includes multiple T-20 programs such as NYU (Grossman), Columbia, Mount Sinai (Icahn), and Cornell (Weill). If I was following my own advice, then I should have applied to all programs including these T-20 schools. As a 510 MCAT scorer, I had to be realistic and come to terms with the fact that these 520+ average MCAT programs would never consider me. I would have been throwing money into the wind or better yet paying the postage for my own rejection letter. As a rule of thumb when considering your state schools, you can extend your Reach School range to +6 points. For me, this would expand my spreadsheet to 516 but only for programs in New York. If you are going to gamble on reach schools, your home-state has the best odds, particularly state schools more so than private programs.

Another interesting way to take advantage of home-state preference is to change your legal residence. Many of you attended or are currently attending pharmacy schools outside of your home state. Considering our 6–8-year pharmacy school commitment, you may be eligible to change your legal residence. I am from New York, but I went to pharmacy school in Pennsylvania. During my tenure in pharmacy school, I had an apartment, paid utilities, and worked a job. All of these features made me eligible to apply for a Pennsylvania driver's license and change my legal residence. Note that every state will have different qualifications but changing your legal address may benefit you during the application cycle. By doing so, you may be able to take advantage of home-state preference or qualify for in-state tuition which is far cheaper than out-of-state. Considering I was from New York, one of the few states with 10+ medical schools, I elected not to change my address. As the reader, you may not be as fortunate being from states with only 1-2 programs. Perhaps you are from a state without a single medical school like Delaware, Montana, Alaska, or Wyoming. Keep in mind that this option is NOT for everyone. It will benefit students who attend pharmacy schools in states with a large quantity of medical schools and programs that provide heavy home-state preference. The following example should clarify the benefits of changing your legal address. A California resident with a 509 MCAT and a 3.67 total GPA attends pharmacy school in Pennsylvania. They qualify to change their legal address after PY2 year, and they do so with the intent of applying to medical school in the future. This was a strategic play because statistically speaking California applicants are a "dime a dozen." Coming from a state with a population of approximately 40 million residents, there are more California applicants than almost any other state. The sheer fact that there are substantially more applicants ultimately raises the talent pool statistics and makes attending a California based medical school that much harder to get into. In short, by reclassifying as a Pennsylvania resident, our student is more likely to benefit from the home-state preference when compared to their birth-state of California. Additionally, some medical schools will want you to be a resident for a particular period of time before you qualify. Keep this in mind as making the switch 6 months before you apply may not be as practical compared to doing so 2 years ahead.

If the home-state preference hasn't convinced you to wait in line at the DMV, then consider the tuition benefits of a future acceptance. There are downsides to changing your legal residence including costs incurred and the time needed to research the switch. I can't speak from experience, but I wanted to introduce this particular application strategy niche.

LOW-YIELD PROGRAMS:

Our next topic of discussion concerns Low-Yield Programs (LYPs). This designation refers to programs that receive over 10,000 applications every cycle or have an extremely small medical school class size (< 60 students). Once again you are playing a numbers game. Most medical schools only have time for a specific number of interviews each cycle and it typically ranges from 400-1,000 per cycle. If "Program A" only receives 5,000 applicants and interviews 500 students a cycle, you have a 10% chance of getting an interview. Conversely, "Program B" receives 12,000 applications and only offers 700 interviews. Program B has afforded applicants a 5.8% chance of getting an interview. Keep in mind we are only talking about interviews here. Realistically, only $1/3^{rd}$ of those who interview will get accepted. The only benefit of LYPs is that they tend to matriculate a lot of out-of-state applicants, eliminating home-state preference bias. Considering that most applicants will meet the qualifications for MCAT and GPA, you should still apply to LYPs if you have the financial means. You can't win the lottery if you don't purchase a ticket! I put this section here to highlight the importance of recognizing these LYPs so that you don't confuse a long application list with having a good one. Some examples of classic LYPs include, Temple, Drexel, Tufts, Georgetown, George Washington, Boston University, Jefferson and more! Look through the MSAR and designate in your google spreadsheet which programs are LYPs.

SCHOOL MISSION:

A medical school's mission statement can reveal what is important to them and how valuable certain aspects of your application will be. This factor will be far more important when writing secondary applications, but it may also help you limit what programs you choose to apply to. There are several main mission archetypes. These include research focused, primary care focused, public or global health oriented, and community service focused. Each medical school will have a unique mission that is typically a hybrid combination of each archetype. Your job is to interpret what each program cares about and see if you have the same qualifications to meet their particular requirements. For example, if you are planning on applying to a top research medical school, you better have extensive research experience including publications and posters presentations. If you are interested in primary care, then you can use this interest of yours to your advantage and select programs that value family medicine. This concept is rather intuitive but another way to fine tune your school list. Understanding a program's mission will also be helpful during secondary writing and critical for a successful interview.

DISTANCE FROM HOME:

This is another important factor that is often overlooked. There is no need to apply to every program in the country, especially if by doing so you end up at a medical school across the country. This can be particularly difficult if you are away from friends and family during another major transition in your life.

If you do not limit your medical school list to programs in a particular region you may be setting yourself up for an extremely expensive interview season. While it is certainly wonderful to get an interview invite the sheer distance and duration of travel can be quite detrimental. You need to remember that you will be on APPE rotations during the interview season and sneaking away for a few days can make your rotation lifestyle cumbersome. While most preceptors understand your unique circumstances, they also have a responsibility to uphold your rotation hour requirements. You may find yourself having to miss a weeks' worth of rotation due to multiple interviews.

In order to accommodate multiple interviews, you may find yourself having to participate in extra rotation assignments or extending your daily hours to pack everything in. Interviews can be offered at any point of the week and each one will typically require 2 days off, especially if you need to travel far. Keep this in mind if you plan on applying to programs all over the country. You may even find yourself traveling across the country several times if your interview slots are poorly matched up. The further away you have to travel, the greater your air-fare expenses will be. It would be much cheaper to drive to the medical school the night before the interview than it would be to fly across the country.

To avoid putting yourself in this position, limit yourself to one region if possible. For instance, I only applied to east coast programs. I excluded any program in the Midwest or beyond. Subsequently, I was able to drive to every interview and avoid most travel costs (baggage fees, food, and drink, etc.) By avoiding distant programs, you have now placed an additional filter on your school list. At this point in time, your list has probably begun to shrink to a manageable and comprehensible size.

COST OF TUITION:

As we begin to finalize your medical school list there is one last consideration to factor in, that being the cost of attendance. Cost of tuition has <u>no</u> impact on your chances of getting accepted and is therefore the <u>least important</u> factor when it comes to making a strong school list. However, it ironically is the most important factor concerning your future financial health. **While I do not recommend you exclude a program from your list solely on the cost of tuition, I want to you be aware of the costliest medical schools.**

PHARM.D. TO M.D.

U.S. News recently published an article concerning the top 10 most expensive medical schools. You can find the article posted in the references below. I have provided a chart from the article demonstrating the astronomically high costs of a medical school education. Note how this is only the cost of ONE YEAR of schooling. Multiply it by 4 and you will be sitting just shy of $300,000 in loans. What nauseates me the most is that this is only the baseline fee to walk the hallways at these institutions. These calculations exclude costs of living so feel free to add another 50-100 grand to your loan burden! As a reminder, you may also have a six-figure pharmacy school loan balance, lest you forget. Alternatively, U.S. News also provided a list of the cheapest medical schools for out-of-state matriculants. Please do not avoid applying to a program for financial reasons but it is an important consideration to make down the road when you must choose between two acceptances. We will touch on this more in future chapters.

Most Expensive		Most Affordable	
School	Tuition Cost/Year	School	Tuition Cost/Year
Midwestern University (IL)	$74,035	University of Cincinnati	$51,133
Midwestern University (AZ)	$71,833	University of Florida	$49,538
Columbia University (NY)	$71,107	University of New Mexico	$48,608
Brown University (RI)	$70,425	Ohio State University	$42,795
Case Western Reserve University (OH)	$70,339	University of Texas Health Science Center – San Antonio	$36,671
Northwestern University (IL)	$70,254	SUNY Upstate Medical University (NY)	$36,196
Dartmouth College (NH)	$69,768	University of North Texas Health Science Center	$35,174
University of Southern California	$69,237	University of Texas Southwestern Medical Center	$34,390
Washington University in St. Louis (MO)	$68,480	Texas A&M University	$32,824
Georgetown University (DC)	$67,875	Texas Tech University Health Sciences Center	$31,908

- **Resource:** U.S. News Most Expensive Medical Schools: https://www.usnews.com/education/best-graduate-schools/the-short-list-grad-school/articles/most-expensive-private-medical-schools

- **Resource:** U.S. News Cheapest Medical Schools https://www.usnews.com/education/best-graduate-schools/the-short-list-grad-school/articles/most-affordable-medical-schools-for-out-of-state-students

COSTS PER SCHOOL:

Now that you have a comprehensive medical school list, you need to decide how many programs you are going to choose and how much it will cost. Since we are already on the topic of finance, we will start with the costs. When you submit your primary application, you will be charged a fee of $170 for the first medical school, and then an additional $42 for each additional school on your list. If you are applying to 21 allopathic programs this will set, you back $1,010. This cost soon multiplies after factoring in secondary application fees. For more information on total costs for applying to medical school, check out the AAMC link below. Additionally, I recommend you play around with this Medical School Headquarters' **Application Cost Estimator**. It will help put everything into perspective and give you a reasonable estimate for the application cycle price tag.

- **Resource:** AAMC Cost of Applying to Medical School: https://students-residents.aamc.org/financial-aid-resources/cost-applying-medical-school

- **Resource:** Medical School HQ Application Cost Estimator https://medicalschoolhq.net/medical-school-applications-cost-estimator/

HOW MANY SCHOOLS SHOULD YOU APPLY TO:

According to Shemassian Academic Consulting, the average number of medical schools' students apply to is 16 programs. Realistically, you should aim for approximately 20-30 programs. If you have already created a "smart" list of schools, then applying to more programs will bolster your chances of getting accepted. As a caveat, you run the risk of burning out mentally and financially from an endless onslaught of secondary applications that will fill your inbox. Some argue that applying to too many schools leads to a deterioration of secondary writing quality. While this may be true to some extent, it can be easily avoided with proper and efficient pre-writing. As you know I applied to 34 programs and it was a massive undertaking, especially while on APPE rotations. Was I miserable? Absolutely! Would I do it again? Without a doubt! At the end of the day, applying to more programs and the subsequent increase in workload is but a small burden when the alternative is having to re-apply next cycle! Pick the lesser of two evils and strap-in for a grueling month of writing.

When determining how many programs you want to apply to, it is imperative that you also consider the distribution model that we discussed. For example, "Student-Z" has decided they want to apply to 30 programs for this application cycle. While they have a high quantity of programs on their list, it turns out that of those 30 programs, 23 of them were Student-Z's reach schools. Student-Z is going to struggle during the cycle and will likely need to re-apply the following year. It is critical for an applicant to be realistic about their application health and to apply with a smart school list.

As a final note, you are able to add programs even after you submit your final AMCAS. If you are unsure about a particular school, you can easily resubmit your AMCAS and they will distribute your application to the newly added school! I found myself adding programs for several weeks post-submission because I had a poorly crafted school list. Hopefully after reading this book, you won't have to worry about adding missed programs.

TAKEAWAYS:

- Create a smart-medical school list utilizing the distribution categories, Safety, Target, and Reach Schools.

- Use your MCAT score to establish a range of programs to apply to.

- Be aware of in-state/out-of-state bias, a useful or hurtful reality depending on your legal residence.

- Watch out for low-yield programs that will sneak onto your school list due to their attainable average MCAT scores.

- Review each programs school mission and adjust your list based on whether or not you would be a good fit.

- Narrow down your list to a particular region if possible, to save money and time during interview season.

- DO NOT let the cost of a school's tuition scare you away from applying. That information will be used to discern between two acceptances later on.
- Your primary application is $170 dollars for the first school and $42 for every additional school that you add to your application.

- Apply to 20-30 medical schools to maximize your chances of getting accepted somewhere.

THE PERSONAL STATEMENT:

This is arguably the most important part of your primary application. Your personal statement essay is the first real opportunity the admissions committee will have to find out who you really are. A strong personal statement will be the cornerstone of your application, and some interviewers will ONLY review this essay. Therefore, this is your personal constitution, a literary work designed to paint a mental picture of your identity to help a future reviewer understand why you want to be a physician. This is no easy task and often requires months of writing and re-writing before you create the final product. I recommend that you begin writing this throughout your PY3 year, especially if you have already conquered the MCAT. Finding the motivation and inspiration to write this beast of an essay is no easy task. Generally speaking, you will need to choose a topic or theme and let that concept tie your essay together like a novel. The hardest part about this process is determining what that topic will be. Remember, when it comes to crafting this personal mission statement, there are no bad ideas. However, there is such a thing as poor execution. Poorly articulated essays can make you look like a cookie-cutter applicant with a cliché write-up. As a pharmacy student, your personal statement already has a foundational concept that needs to be addressed. You will need to discuss why you are making such a drastic career switch! Already an excellent starting point with a unique twist. You will need to personalize this concept as you go and make the idea your own. You may even have a better and more character-revealing story to share so don't let me discourage you from writing about it either! Let's dive into the writing process to see what it takes to create a world class personal statement.

HOW TO WRITE YOUR PERSONAL STATEMENT:

The AMCAS Applicant Guide recommends that as an applicant, you explain why you selected medicine, what motivates you to continue this pursuit, and what unique hardships, challenges, or obstacles you may have faced along the way. While this can be a good way to start, they hardly address how to really create a poetic work. The only real pointer they provide is the character limit which is a measly 5,300 characters. At least you have some limitations to your memoir, so don't feel like you have to write an autobiography. According to Shemmassian Academic Counseling, there are three easy steps to drafting a strong personal statement.

#1: List your greatest qualities. This would include features that describe your character, personality traits, and attitudes about medicine and life in general. Some examples include extraordinary, compassionate, kind, optimistic, persistent, steadfast, creative, and so on. Create your own list that you think represents you.

#2: When have you demonstrated these qualities? Fill in your list of words with supporting detail to prove that you are who you say you are. If you are truly compassionate, then talk about the time you took care of your sick aunt, made a clinically impactful medication change, or made someone's day while volunteering. These qualities don't even need to be reinforced with clinical experiences and should be supported by stories that represent the real you.

#3: Describe your event as a story. Adding yet another layer of complexity, utilize your variety of stories and craft them into a logical storyboard. You want your future reader to be engaged so make your story sound like an adventure. The last thing you want is a bland essay that rocks your reader to sleep.

#4: Discuss how your experiences have led you down the path to medicine. For example, "at first I started volunteering in the hospital as a high school student then fell in love with healthcare. I attended pharmacy school but realized that I could do so much more for patients by utilizing this specialized knowledge as a physician." Your own version will have to be far more poetic than this short example, but you can use it as a starting point! I also recommend you make a chronological bulleted list of your journey into medicine. Having a template can help you avoid missing important details and provide a framework to guide you along the way.

One of the biggest mistakes that students make when writing their personal statement is that they use the essay as a way to boast about their achievements. **They talk about things that they think will impress an admissions committee and they often miss the entire point of the personal statement.** While it may be fun to talk about how great you did in pharmacy school or even high school, don't. This is your opportunity to demonstrate humility, a time that medicine changed you, or how your experiences have impacted the course of your life. This is certainly not the time to talk about how smart you are, how you got a 4.0 in school, or won an award. The admissions committee knows you are qualified. You have already proven that in the rest of your primary application. They want to see that you are human, that you make mistakes, and that you can overcome them in a positive and productive manner.

This is also NOT the time to discuss how you disliked pharmacy and that was the reason for your switch. Notice the difference in tone. It sounds way better to describe your switch as the "next step on your journey" than to talk about how "wrong pharmacy was for you personally." While that is certainly not the story for everyone reading this book, it shouldn't even come up when writing your personal statement. **Positive experiences trump negative ones so please don't bash the very same profession that has gotten you to the threshold of becoming a physician.** You have likely been proclaiming how important your pharmacy experiences have been, so do not undermine them here. Better yet, use your background as leverage to add some flavor to your personal statement. Make your reader love pharmacy school and talk about how influential it was to you. You would be lying if you didn't!

PERSONAL STATEMENT EDITING:

This section may seem rather intuitive, but you'd be surprised how many applicants disregard a second opinion. I get it, your personal statement is a testament to who you are, and you may feel self-conscious of the quality (especially after putting in hundreds of hours of work into this manifesto). **I cannot stress this enough – you need to have others read and edit your work.** You should also get a variety of people to look it over. While it may be nice to have your mother read it through, she may not be the most constructive or realistic when reading your work. The last thing you need is for your editor to "sugar-coat" the bad news, being that your essay is substandard, or just plain sucks. Outside input can resolve typos or help fix the underlying structure of your essay. I recommend you get several reviewers with a variety of experience to comb through your work, sentence by sentence. I have listed a few editors that you should inquire about finding below.

#1: A Family Member: This is someone who has known you for a long time and can relate to the personal components of your essay. You share a relationship with this editor so they will be able to understand the particular angle you take. They will also serve as a morale booster!

#2: A Harsh Critic: This individual will likely be a pharmacy school professor, physician, or professional mentor. They will offer you a realistic and objective take on the quality of your work. Having someone in academia can be particularly useful because of their expertise. While the feedback may strike at your ego, you should internalize the comments and create a stronger essay.

#3: A Grammar Freak: This editor will forgo the content of the essay, and scrutinize the sentence structure, formatting, and punctuation. This is a vital component when drafting a logical and well-versed essay. Your university likely has a writing center that should grant you access to a professional review. I went to my university's writing center and had several graduate students in English revise my work. While you may be an expert on the top 200 prescribed drugs, you are probably underqualified to write. Use some professional guidance along the way to make this process so much easier!

#4: A Stranger: While your grammar freak may fill this slot as well, they are likely only focused on the punctation. Finding an absolute stranger can provide you with unbiased criticism. See how well your essay tells your life story and if your reader can grasp the main idea. Remember, your future reviewer will also be a complete stranger too!

Now that you had a second set of eyes look over your content, you will have to choose which advise you should use. While it may be nice to have outside opinions, some suggestions may not be in your best interest. Don't heed any advice that you think will subtract meaning from the essay, or anything that you think obstructs a reader's interpretation. In the end, this is your journey and your reflection so make sure at the end of the criticism, it still represents you! If you are interested in more information, check out this excellent post from a fellow reddit student below discussing the intricacies of writing a personal statement. Their post served as the inspiration for this particular section.

- **Resource:** Writing A Personal Statement: Reddit
  https://www.reddit.com/r/premed/comments/fh3s2y/writing_your_personal_statement_a_howto/

PART FIVE:

SECONDARY APPLICATIONS

"If you set your goal ridiculously high and it's a failure, you will fail above everyone else's success"

– James Cameron

Congratulations, if you are reading this you have officially submitted your primary application. You are almost through the most difficult months of the application cycle and are that much closer to getting into medical school! Secondary applications are just like they sound: more writing and tedious work required by almost every medical school. I know, right! When is this guy going give me some good news? Secondary applications are yet another way for medical schools to learn about who you are but with an added twist. They will ask you why you are interested in their particular program or give you the opportunity to reflect upon challenges you have faced. In my humble and <u>personal opinion</u>, secondary applications are just another money-grab opportunity for medical schools to take cash from distressed applicants. You're going to tell me that these institutions need $130 to read my 3 poorly written paragraphs about how great the medical school program is. Yeah, sure that seems reasonable! Anyways, no sense in complaining because like it or not it's a requirement.

SECONDARY OVERVIEW:

In short, secondary applications are a way each individual medical school can ask you specific questions that are not seen on your primary application. Historically, getting a secondary application meant that the program of interest was piqued by your primary application, and they wanted to get more information before offering you an interview seat. What was once considered a small achievement is now just another hoop for you to jump through. **Most medical schools will automatically send you a secondary application before they even screen your application.** In other words, save your excitement for the interview offer. You can find out which programs provide automatic secondary requests through the MSAR or by reviewing each program's personal website. Programs that automatically send secondary applications include, Howard, Loyola Chicago, NYU, Penn State, Stanford, SUNY Upstate, Marshall, Morehouse, Michigan State, and Mount Sinai just to list a few.

Writing secondary application essays can be quite challenging especially with the sheer volume of applications. Depending on how many medical schools you decided to send your primary application to, you should expect to get a secondary application from almost everyone. There are still programs out there that will screen you out if you do not meet their GPA or MCAT standards.

Within each secondary you will come across anywhere from 1-10 essay prompts with an average count of 3-4. For a student who applied to 25 schools you can expect to write close to 100 individual prompts. Yikes! To further complicate things, you are racing against the clock to get your secondary applications completed. Some programs request completed documents within 2 weeks of notification. Others don't provide a deadline which can be just as difficult without external motivators to push you to completion. Most medical schools that send you a secondary application will not consider you eligible for review until you have finished all the submittable work. Therefore, a student who completes the secondary application sooner will be reviewed first and have a better chance of getting a limited number of interview invites. Of course, this is pending the submission of additional requirements including your Casper exam scores and more. **Despite how quickly you want to submit your secondary application, the quality of the work should take priority.** Avoid the temptation to submit a poorly written secondary just for the sake of getting it complete. You are so close to being done with the hardest 2 months of the application cycle, so finish strong! In order to avoid a mental breakdown, I *strongly* encourage you to pre-write your prompts.

PRE-WRITE YOUR SECONDARY APPLICATIONS:

While each medical school can choose to ask you anything, they tend to fall into specific categories. This includes essay prompts, asking you about challenges you have overcome, diversity/inclusion topics, community service-oriented, and the reasons for wanting to go to a particular medical school. These particular essays can be pre-written and then retrofitted to meet the specific requests of each medical school. After a few minor adjustments, you will be able to submit your secondary application within a few hours of getting your notification. Excellent turnaround time gets your application to the finish line and hopefully ready for an interview offer.

So how do you pre-write? Fortunately, most medical schools will reuse the same prompts from year-to-year. You should be able to find the prompts with a quick Google search. Alternatively, you can find prompts at **Prospective Doctor's** website. Some programs will change their essay questions every couple years so be prepared to scrap some pre-written essays! If you are crunched on time, I recommend you pre-write the essays for the programs you are most interested in or have the best chances of getting an acceptance at. Don't spend hundreds of hours crafting the perfect secondary application prompts for your reach schools when you realistically only have a 1-2% chance of even getting an interview.

When writing your essay prompts you can also use some of the content you submitted on your primary application. While it is best to showcase new material that will reveal more of your personality, you may end up with writers-block. If this happens to you, it's generally acceptable to reuse some experiences. Do not just copy and paste your primary application write-ups. Discuss the experience from a different perspective that can address a different lesson you learned or share an important detail that you left out due to character limits. Keep in mind that some programs may specifically ask you for new experiences so pay attention to the fine print.

- **Resource:** Prospective Doctor Secondary Prompt Database: https://www.prospectivedoctor.com/medical-school-secondary-essay-prompts-database/

COMMON SECONDARY PROMPTS:

If you do heed my advice and plan on pre-writing your secondaries, it's important that you address the most commonly asked questions first. A few well-written answers to these questions can be used and reused for multiple applications, saving you plenty of time. Some of these questions are provided below with some potential answers/tips to answering them!

#1: *"Is there a unique aspect of your application that you would like to share with the admissions committee?"*

This is a great opportunity to discuss your unique education and training and how it will contribute to academic excellence and compassionate medical care. Were you participating in the COVID-19 Pandemic Vaccination effort? If so, this would be a great opportunity to share this unique experience with an admission's team.

#2: *"What are your plans leading up to medical school matriculation?"*

Talk about the incredible rotations you will be participating in. Discuss attending future national pharmacy conferences like the ASHP Midyear Clinical Meeting and how you are presenting your research. Discuss how you will be working a full-time job in a pharmacy during your off-blocks or how you plan to use that time to shadow more physicians. Medical schools want to see that you are staying busy and continuing to build your skills, even after you have submitted the vast majority of your application content.

#3: *"Why did you apply to our school?"*

"XYZ School of Medicine has excellent medical facilities, a cutting-edge curriculum, and a devout passion for patient care demonstrated by *insert amazing club or organization*. These qualities are exactly what I am looking for in a medical school. My experiences with *insert life changing patient encounter* have prepared me to be a professional and compassionate medical provider. Because of *insert more amazing experiences*, I would be a great fit for this program."

Pay close attention to how you craft this essay. When writing these it's very easy to talk about all the great programs, clubs, and academics a program has to offer. By doing so exclusively, you will make your essay cliché and quite frankly boring. The admissions committee already knows how amazing their medical school is, trust me when I say you don't need to remind them. **What they want to know is how YOUR experiences fit into the culture of the institution. They want to know what YOU could contribute and how you can grow these programs.** Introduce an idea that can improve a club or something that can benefit current or future students. For example, if you went on a medical mission trip to a particular country, introduce the idea of setting up a similar trip at the institution. Express your passion for global health through action. You could also talk about building a collaborative practice club that allows medical students to work with pharmacy students, nurses, physician assistants and so on to solve case-based problems. You could offer to use your pharmacy knowledge to create a drug-based resource to help future medical students who often struggle with pharmacology. My point is that you need to avoid the cookie-cutter responses and show that you are not only a good fit for the program, but that you will actively contribute once you get in.

#4: *"Describe a personal challenge and how you overcame it."*

This answer will have to be something personal and unique to you. I can't give you a perfect answer here, but the general idea should focus on an experience you had that was difficult or stressful. Medical schools want to see how you managed the adversity, how you attempted to resolve the issue at hand, and if you can appropriately reflect on the experience. Lastly, they want to see if you learned from the experience and can apply those principles to future challenges. This is not meant to be a competition to show off how much you suffered. Rather, how you overcame difficult circumstances in life regarding relationships, family, medical issues, major criticism, and more.

#5: *"How will you enhance our school's diversity?"*

To answer this question you will need to express awareness of diverse health beliefs, practices, needs, and accessibility to care. You must also demonstrate that you have a willingness to understand these differences and that you will be use this understanding to better serve patients as a physician. The great thing about being in pharmacy school is you will have already worked with a variety of different patient populations and should be able to reflect upon some unique interactions. You may also want to focus on other important events such as a medical mission trip, experience/understanding of health disparities, or your multicultural competency.

#6: *"Is there anything else you'd like us to know about you?"*

This is a freelance essay that you can use to share any unique feature about yourself. Depending on the other questions you are asked in a particular secondary application, you may want to talk about pharmacy, a hobby you have, an incredible patient encounter, your passion for research, or how you would be an excellent fit for their program. **This essay prompt is sometimes "optional" but in my opinion, always mandatory.** If a medical school gives you more real estate to build up your application, do it! This will be the last way to communicate with most medical schools prior to a thorough inspection of your submitted content.

#7: *"Where do you see yourself in 10-years?"*

This essay prompt is not as common, but it should come up several times during your cycle. It has also come up in interviews so having a solid and thoughtful response can be useful even after you submit your secondary application. If you are passionate about a particular medical specialty discuss that here. Make sure you back up your reasoning from experience, such as a beneficial rotation that exposed you to the field or from a positive shadowing experience. If you aren't sure about a career field yet, don't sweat it! Medical schools know that your future profession will change 10-times throughout your medical school tenure. Instead of talking about a profession, talk about what kind of doctor you want to be from a quality standpoint. "In 10-years I want to be a doctor that is empathetic, a strong communicator, understanding, respectful of different opinions and beliefs, knowledgeable, and professional." You can discuss how you want to become an associate professor and give back to student education, advance research directives, or just plain have a family and give back to the community. This essay is what you make of it. The key is that you demonstrate that you are driven, that you hope to improve medicine, and change lives!

SECONDARY ESSAY TIMING:

As we have already mentioned, writing secondaries in a timely manner will give you an advantage with regard to medical school rolling admissions. Not only are you fighting against the clock, but you will need to stick to a rigid schedule to avoid getting bogged down with countless secondaries. If you are able to complete each secondary within several days of receipt, you will be able to stay on top of the content load, a particularly challenging task when balancing your APPE rotations. I remember spending 8 hours on the hospital wards, just learning how to handle my new responsibilities, then getting home and writing essays for 4-5 hours every night. Most applicants will be on summer break or will be taking advantage of a gap year and will have time to lollygag and build stunning essays. You must maintain a schedule and complete little chunks of essay writing each day. If you wait around those 2-3 secondary applications will balloon into 25 and tackling that load of work will seem unapproachable and could lead to burnout. The best method to writing these prompts can be achieved with this simple schedule.

Day 1: Your secondary arrives in your inbox. Read the prompts and see if any fit with your pre-written content. If not, start writing immediately!

Day 2: If you didn't complete the secondary prompts, use this second day to complete the prompts and to reformat content as necessary. One of the most annoying features of secondary application essays is adjusting your writing to fit the character count or word limit. Often times you will have to condense your content and use concise wording to avoid losing meaning in your statements.

Day 3: Now that you have taken some time away from the writing process complete your final proofreading and editing. After taking a break from writing you will have a new sense of clarity that will make typos and poorly articulated points much more obvious. Take the most time with your favorite programs to make sure everything is perfect. Upon approval of your final inspection, submit it and move on to your next secondary application. Rinse and repeat!

This schedule should be effective enough to complete most secondary applications. Don't fret if you need more time but please stay focused and don't get bogged down. There are also secondary applications that are particularly difficult. University of Miami, Duke, and UCLA have notoriously long and difficult secondary essays that take some applicants weeks to complete. Adjust your expectations accordingly and strap in for the long hall.

PART SIX:

THE CASPER EXAM

"A successful individual is one who can lay a firm foundation with the bricks others have thrown at them."

– David Brikley

CASPER (Computer-Based Assessment for Sampling Personal Characteristics) is a situational judgmental assessment that will assess a candidate's professionalism, understanding of ethics, communication skills and empathy. This new examination has only been around for several years and emerged due to the inability for letters of recommendation and personal statement essays to adequately evaluate a candidate's personal characteristics. A new addition to the previous CASPER exam requirements is the **Altus Suite** package. Altus Suite includes the CASPER Exam, SNAPSHOT, and DUET programs, now required for students applying to the 2021-2022 application cycle. Don't freak out just yet though, only about 10 medical schools require SNAPSHOT or DUET at the moment. I anticipate that this list will grow over the years so it may be in your best interest to complete all 3. For other programs not on the list their requirements are somewhat ambiguous stating that Altus Suite is highly recommended.

You may also be wondering how much does this cost? I hope I have trained you well to know that nothing is free, and this is certainly no exception. Fortunately, the Altus Suite only costs $12 to participate and then an additional $12 per medical school that you send your score report to. If you applied to 30 programs, approximately 15-20 of them will require scores, leading to a cost range of $192-$252. I am sure you are starting to see how all of these expenses are adding up very quickly. If you think this is bad, just wait until you see the cost of interviews!

Altus Suite/CASPER Exam are all taken remotely from your own personal device. There is no need to travel to a testing center to complete each of these components. You will need a reliable internet connection, working video camera and audio, and a quite workspace. You will only be able to submit your contents once and you will not have access to any of your submitted responses or videos. This is a one-and-done event, so make sure your family doesn't walk through the background. Disable incoming phone calls if you are taking the exam on a capable device and be sure that you are well-rested!

ALTUS SUITE COMPONENTS:

CASPER:

An online situational judgement test that screens applicants for 10 non-cognitive competencies including ethics, empathy, problem-solving and collaboration. The exam exposes applicants to 12 unique scenarios, 8 of which are video-based, and 4 of which are text-based. For each unique scenario, the applicant will be asked 3 questions related to the situation or may be asked a stand-alone question about their own experiences. The applicant will only have 5 minutes to complete the 3 questions, so fast thinking and quick typing are essential. The applicant will have 60-90 minutes to complete the assessment in total. When responding to short prompts, each student will have several minutes to type out a response. The grading process takes approximately 2-3 weeks, and you will be given a quartile rank. This is a new feature for applicants in the 2021-2022 application cycle. Your quartile is not a representation of how many questions you answered correctly but rather how well you performed relative to your peers.

Most academic programs are incorporating CASPER scores into their admissions processes to better screen students who are academically gifted but socially or ethically deficient. As you all know, medicine is no longer just a "who knows most" business. It involves working with people, far more collaboration with peers, and handling difficult or sensitive situations. Medical schools want students who can do both academics and work with people. In all honesty, most programs are more inclined to take a 512 MCAT scoring applicant with good social skills than a 526 MCAT scorer who hasn't left their house in years.

SCHOOLS REQUIRING CASPER:

This is the current list for the 2021-2022 application cycle of all allopathic medical schools in the U.S. that require the CASPER exam.

Allopathic Medical Schools:
- Augusta University Medical College of Georgia
- Baylor College of Medicine
- Boston University School of Medicine
- Central Michigan University College of Medicine
- Chicago Medical School at Rosalind Franklin University
- Donald and Barbara Zucker School of Medicine at Hofstra/Northwell
- Drexel University College of Medicine
- East Tennessee State University Quillen College of Medicine
- Florida Atlantic University College of Medicine
- Howard University College of Medicine
- Indiana University School of Medicine
- Marshall University Joan C. Edwards School of Medicine
- Medical College of Wisconsin
- Meharry Medical College
- Mercer University School of Medicine
- Michigan State University College of Human Medicine
- New York Medical College
- Northeast Ohio Medical University
- Oregon Health & Sciences University School of Medicine
- Penn State College of Medicine
- Rutgers New Jersey Medical School

PHARM.D. TO M.D.

- Rutgers Robert Wood Johnson Medical School
- Stony Brook University Renaissance School of Medicine
- SUNY Update Medical University
- Temple University Lewis Katz School of Medicine
- Texas A&M University College of Medicine
- Texas Tech University Health Sciences Center
- Tulane University School of Medicine
- University of Colorado School of Medicine
- University of Illinois College of Medicine
- University of Miami Miller School of Medicine
- University of Michigan Medical School
- University of Nevada, Reno School of Medicine
- University of Texas Health Science Center, McGovern Medical School, Long School of Medicine, Galveston School of Medicine
- University of Texas Southwestern Medical School
- University of Vermont Larner College of Medicine
- University of Washington School of Medicine
- Virginia Commonwealth University School of Medicine
- Virginia Tech Carilion School of Medicine
- Wake Forest School of Medicine
- West Virginia University School of Medicine

Osteopathic Medical Schools:

- Alabama College of Osteopathic Medicine
- Arkansas College of Osteopathic Medicine
- California Health Sciences University College of Osteopathic Medicine
- Idaho College of Osteopathic Medicine
- Michigan State University College of Osteopathic Medicine
- Oklahoma State University College of Osteopathic Medicine
- Pacific Northwest University of Health Sciences
- Sam Houston State University College of Osteopathic Medicine
- Touro University Nevada
- Touro College of Osteopathic Medicine (NY)
- Western University of Health Sciences College of Osteopathic Medicine of the Pacific and Pacific-Northwest
- William Carey University College of Osteopathic Medicine

WHEN TO TAKE THE CASPER EXAM:

As mentioned, the CASPER Exam takes approximately 2-3 weeks to receive your final score. Some medical schools require your CASPER score report before they can consider your application complete for review. **In other words, even if you finish your secondary application, they will not review your submitted contents until after they have your CASPER Score.** While this may be the case for some medical schools, others will still review your contents regardless. Considering that CASPER is a newer part of the application process some medical schools technically require it but are using it for data purposes to see how well the scores correlate with the students they traditionally accept.

In general, you should aim to submit your CASPER a couple weeks before you plan on finishing secondary applications. This may be as early as May if you are proactive with the application cycle. Because of my unorganized, and lackadaisical application cycle, I ended up taking my CASPER in early July. I recommend you complete this earlier, if possible, but it won't be the end of the world if it holds you up a few weeks. I was so focused on finishing my primary application while getting adjusted to my first APPE rotation that the CASPER was the last thing on my mind. While my tardiness had no obvious repercussions, the CASPER exam has grown in popularity since I was first tasked with taking it. Some programs are placing more weight on performance and timing as the years go by.

Fortunately, this exam if far simpler than the MCAT and requires at most, 2-3 days of preparation. You can usually sign up quickly, reserve a test date/time, and take the exam all within a few weeks. I recommend you take it as soon as possible to get it out of your way. In the grand scheme of the application cycle, this is an easy box to check-off.

TACKLING THE CASPER EXAM:

Rule number one, "don't be a sociopath. If you are, learn how to hide it." This was a quote from the reddit forum that I could not resist sharing! In all seriousness, there is a formulated method to high performance on the CASPER.

What kind of questions should you expect? The exam will prompt you with either text or videos of ethical, personal, work-related situations that you will have to watch or read then answer a prompt. The caveat is that you have a limited amount of time to respond to the prompts which will ask you to review each scenario. Your 12 certified reviewers will be looking for qualities that demonstrate your values, assess your approach to conflict, and ability to consider different perspectives. The 3 questions you receive per scenario usually ask about how you would handle the situation, ask about specific events in the scenario, or share a similar experience you had relating to the situation. You will not only need to have a method to tackle the questions at hand, but you will need write about relatable situations off the top of your head. We will start with Altus Suite's recommendations which are listed below.

- Start your test without unnecessary worries.

- Take the full five minutes to respond.

- Read fully, then plan your response.

- Don't panic if you don't finish your thought.

- Find a quiet place to take the test.

- Don't bother cheating.

- Be familiar with the format.

- Should I pay for coaching or test prep? I can answer this for you. **Absolutely NOT!** There are online courses that are asking for several thousands of dollars guaranteeing top quartile scores. All they ask for is a diabolical amount of money to train you how to take a common-sense examination.

You can read more about the specifics from Altus Suite but these recommendations are generic and rather useless. I placed them here so that you have the material from the test maker but realistically you will need a proven method with actual instruction on how to do well.

Introducing the PPRDJ Method, which is one of the most popular and successful ways to crush the CAPSER! This gold standard technique stands for **"Problem, Perspective, Responsibility, Decision, Justification (PPRDJ)."** This method is self-explanatory so let's take a look at an example below and apply it to a possible scenario.

"Emily has been showing up to work late for the past few days and her absence has forced some of the other employees to pick up the extra work. You are the supervisor at the company and the disgruntled employees confront you. They are asking that you reprimand Emily for her tardy behavior and consider firing her. How should you respond to this situation?"

Problem: *Emily has been late to work for several days, and her coworkers are upset about doing her share of work.*

Perspective: *I understand why the employees are frustrated with Emily. I agree that doing extra work is not necessarily fair and is not part of their job description. Additionally, I need to confront Emily but in an inquisitive manner. Perhaps, I don't know the entire story. She may be a new hire and her daily start time for her shift was not properly communicated. Alternatively, she may be dealing with personal stressors in her family/home life that I may not know about which could be impacting her ability to show up to work on time.*

Responsibility: *As the supervisor, it is my responsibility to take action to resolve the issue at hand. As a supervisor, I need to be fair to all my employees and hear both sides of the story. Emily's coworkers may have a reasonable argument, but it is important that I consider Emily's perspective. I should gather more information to be sure that all the facts check out.*

Decision/Justification: *After talking with Emily, it turns out that her 5-year-old son has had the flu for the past couple days, and she has been struggling to care for him and come to work. I have decided to offer Emily the opportunity to work from home which is part of the standard practice at our company. I have communicated with the other employees who are understanding of her circumstances and appreciate that she will be able to continue to work.*

There are several other approaches that students can utilize for CASPER exam preparation, but the PPRDJ Method seems to be good enough without overcomplicating things.

CREATE YOUR OWN EXAMPLES:

You will not only have to answer scenario-based questions but there will be a few stand-alone examples asking about a related personal experience. Don't spend too much time working on these (1-2 hours max). It is not like you are going to memorize the material you write word for word anyways. The writing process will help you brainstorm some of the topics and internalize lead ideas. Review them right before you take the exam so that they are fresh in your head. You may also come across a prompt that you haven't pre-written so have 2-3 backup ideas just in case. Pre-write the following examples listed below.

- A time you confronted an authority figure.

- A situation where you had to work with a group or team, and it wasn't going well.

- A time when someone treated you unfairly.

- An instance where you witnessed an unethical situation and how you handled it.

- Think about a time you had to make a sacrifice in order to accomplish a goal.
- A time you were wrong and how you handled it.

SAMPLE QUESTIONS/RESOURCES:

#1: Altus Suite offers several video-based scenario examples. These videos will be very similar to the content on the actual exam. What AAMC content is to the MCAT, Altus Suite content is to the CASPER. I worked through several of the videos myself when I was preparing for the exam and felt more comfortable on test day.

- **Resource**: Altus Suite Example Problems
  https://takealtus.com/test-prep/

#2: Another excellent resource includes **Astroff Consultants** who have put together additional content to practice with. They offer 1 video-based example and 9 text-based scenarios. Other than these two resources you shouldn't need much more practice! If for some reason you do, there are plenty of other resources available online.

- **Resource**: Astroff Consultants
  https://www.caspertest.com/casper-sample-questions/

CASPER EXAM SUMMARY:

- There are 12 scenarios. You have 5 minutes to answer 3 questions for each scenario.

- Sign up as soon as possible to avoid application delays. Ideally before secondary applications are posted.

- Memorize the PPDRJ Method, practice the approach with multiple examples or free online content.

- Approach each scenario in a non-judgmental manner, **make no assumptions about someone's behavior**, demonstrate understanding, and analyze both perspectives in a conflict.

- Pre-write situational experiences involving yourself, that can be easily adapted to fit several situations.

- Preparation time should not exceed 2-3 days. Anything more is overkill.

- Work quickly, and don't get side-tracked. Don't concern yourself with spelling or punctuation. These errors will not count against you unless the final product is practically illegible.

SNAPSHOT:

This is a short, one-way video interview to highlight your communication skills and motivation for the profession so you can bring your personal statement to life. It consists of 3 questions which are structured like an actual interview. You will be given a 30 second reflection period to read the question and then 2 minutes of recorded response time. In total the experience only takes 10-15 minutes. You can take this portion of Altus Suite at any point after making your CASPER exam reservation, up until medical school specific deadlines.

Treat this like a formal interview. That means you will need to harbor professional dress, wear neutral colors, avoid fidgeting, maintain good posture, and be conscientious about your body language. This will be the first time that medical schools will see your face, so make sure you provide them with a professional recording that will show your maturity, enthusiasm for medicine, individual personality, and confidence in your ability.

I don't anticipate this being an issue for most pharmacy students who have likely already been on multiple job interviews and have had much more life experience than most traditional applicants. You will find that graduate school has prepared you well for situations like these. While SNAPSHOT is a new feature to the application cycle, I believe it will be another great way to make pharmacy students stand out. While it may be tedious to complete this task, I think it will benefit our niche of applicants in the long run.

PHARM.D. TO M.D.

SNAPSHOT QUESTIONS:

Most questions are related to getting to know you better, particularly about your character as an individual, motivations concerning medicine, and ability to collaborate with others. You can consider this a "Pre-interview" that an admission's committee will review. It is much easier from an admission's standpoint to judge an applicant's demeanor through video than it is through your text-based primary application. SNAPSHOT is only utilized by individual medical schools and is NOT scored by Altus Suite. Some example questions are listed below.

- Tell us about someone you admire and why.

- What is your favorite book? *(Hint, "Pharm.D. to M.D.")*

- What is an obstacle you have faced, and how did you get through it?

- What aspect of your future profession are you most excited about?

While it may be useful to pre-write these listed questions, in all likelihood, you will be asked very different material. Your time will be better spent thinking of life experiences that you can utilize for a variety of different questions. For example, if you worked with a patient in the pharmacy to resolve a prior authorization issue, this could be written up as a meaningful experience, conflict resolution, compassionate care, or even a minor reason for pursing medicine. Your examples must be highly adaptable because it is difficult to predict the exact questions you will be asked. The last thing you need is to internalize a pre-written script and sound mechanical in your interview. Your responses will need to be authentic and thought provoking while successfully answering the prompt. You will need to get good at this for real interviews, so why not start now? For more potential questions you should read through the **500 Interview Question Document** to at least get an idea of what you are up against.

- **Resource**: 500 Interview Question Document
  https://docs.google.com/document/d/1aoaPVqFKXJZjfoqK5wXp
  KFDmqj4hhFwJQOPQ0crHqc8/mobilebasic?utm_source=share
  &utm_medium=ios_app

DUET:

This is a value-alignment assessment that compares what you value in a program with what the program has to offer. Each medical school's characteristics are compared within several different categories with your own. There is no outside preparation required to complete this portion of Altus Suite. You will have unlimited time, but realistically it will only take about 15 minutes. The characteristics that you will come across can be classified under Teaching & Learning, Mission & Culture, and Program Features. Fill out the form and select the characteristics that are most important to you. Remember, there is no correct answer so don't stress too much. Following the same requirements for SNAPSHOT, this portion can be completed as soon as you have a CASPER exam reservation and is available up until the distribution deadline.

AAMC SITUATIONAL JUDGMENT TEST (SJT):

I'd like to introduce Altus Suite's competition, and it's called bureaucracy. The SJT is a new judgement test introduced by the AAMC for the 2021-2022 application cycle. It is very similar to the CASPER exam except that the applicant taking the test will select standardized responses to text-based scenarios instead of typing out essays. After a scenario, the applicant will be tasked with rating particular behaviors with a 4-point scale: 1 = very ineffective, 2 = ineffective, 3 = effective, 4 = very effective. There are 30 scenarios with a total of 186 behaviors that must be rated. The exam runs for approximately 75 minutes, and you can complete it from your home device. For more information about the exam itself and different practice materials you can visit the comprehensive reddit forum designed for the SJT.

The test is currently free although this is subject to change for future test takers. This is likely because the SJT has only been adopted by two medical schools: Morehouse School of Medicine, and University of Alabama Birmingham School of Medicine. There are four others that the SJT is not required but is "STRONGLY recommended." These include Geisinger Commonwealth School of Medicine, University of Minnesota School of Medicine, University of California Davis School of Medicine, and Des Moines University Medicine and Health Sciences. I anticipate that this list will grow larger as the years progress. For the most up to date list of medical schools that require the SJT, you can visit the **AAMC SJT Website**.

- **Resource**: SJT Reddit Forum
  https://www.reddit.com/r/premed/wiki/sjt/

- **Resource**: AAMC SJT Website
  https://students-residents.aamc.org/aamc-situational-judgment-test/participating-medical-schools

TAKEAWAYS:

- The CASPER Exam and the Altus Suite Components SNAPSHOT and DUET are another steppingstone in the application process.

- SNAPSHOT is your first "mini-interview," so treat it like the real-deal.

- DUET is a short 15-minute questionnaire that will help match you to a medical school.

- AAMC SJT is gaining momentum and may replace the Altus Suite package in the coming years.

- You only have to take the Altus Suite package or AAMC SJT if you are applying to programs that require one or the other.

PART SEVEN:

OSTEOPATHIC SCHOOLS OF MEDICINE

"You treat a disease: You win or lose. You treat a person, and I guarantee you win - no matter the outcome."

– Patch Adams

Congratulations, you are on the horizon of finishing the active portion of the application cycle. While interviews afford their own challenges, you are almost through the hardest part of the cycle. You have completed your MCAT, submitted your AMCAS, selected your allopathic schools of medicine, finished secondary applications, and crushed the Altus Suite. Yet another difficult decision to make moving forward involves deciding if you are going to apply to osteopathic medical schools. In general, osteopathic medical schools have slightly lower entry requirements which makes them appealing to applicants with lower medical school statistics (MCAT, GPA, etc.). In recent years, this gap has narrowed as more and more qualified applicants enter the application cycle despite the stagnant number of available seats. Students who would have easily gotten into an allopathic school of medicine 10 years ago, are finding themselves only getting into osteopathic medical programs. The interesting fact is that it's actually harder to get into osteopathic schools based on pure statistics. There are far more allopathic medical schools than osteopathic programs, and subsequently more students matriculate into M.D. schools. From an academic standpoint this statement can be reversed. Check out the American Association for Colleges of Osteopathic Medicine's (AACOM) website for additional information concerning osteopathic medicine.

OSTEOPATHIC PHYSICIAN OVERVIEW:

Students seeking an osteopathic education undergo the same medical school education except for additional modules concerning osteopathic manipulation. This is one of the profession's core philosophies that employs various techniques and movements to heal the human body. A graduate from one these medical schools will receive a Doctorate in Osteopathic Medicine with "D.O." medical credentials. These physicians are licensed to practice medicine in all 50-states and are equivalent to their allopathic (M.D.) counterparts.

Osteopathic physicians are trained to treat patients holistically, and to look for factors beyond a patient's physical ailment. A particularly enticing education for students interested in learning more about natural medicine. Instead of giving a patient a prescription pill, osteopathic physicians focus on manipulation techniques and consider outside variables as contributing factors to disease. Many graduates from these programs are interested in primary care medicine or rural community medicine. If you are also one of these applicants, then applying to a D.O. program would be great for you! Alternatively, if you have ambitions to contribute to massive clinical trials, or practice at the nation's most prestigious medical institutions, an education in osteopathic medicine may not be best for you.

Regardless of what an applicant wants, D.O. programs are of interest because it affords applicants with lower statistics the opportunity to get into medical school instead of taking a gap year.

OSTEOPATHIC MEDICINE LIMITATIONS:

Now that you have a better understanding of this profession, you should be aware of some known disadvantages of seeking an osteopathic education. These limitations are in the context of comparing the education, salary, and future residency opportunities, to allopathic medical students.

#1: Residency Match Rates. One of the most important facets of becoming a physician, if not the most important, is matching into your desired subset of medicine. The whole reason you are committing your heart and soul to this application process is because you want to practice medicine in a particular field that fascinates you. The good news is that the match rates between M.D. and D.O. medical graduates are essentially the same, 92.8% to 89.1%, respectively. The bad news is that statistically speaking, D.O. graduates will have a more difficult time matching into traditionally competitive residency programs. This may also be the case for top-residency programs across the country. While this discrepancy has been in decline for decades now, there are still residency programs that will take preference for M.D. applicants. The chart below is a compilation of the **2021 residency match data** provided by the National Resident Matching Program (NRMP). You may also notice that osteopathic physicians have excellent match rates in less competitive specialties including Emergency Medicine (77.3%), Family Medicine (75.3%), and Internal Medicine (77.4%). Part of this is due to the lower number of M.D. physicians applying to these programs, due to the pursuit of specialty programs. Below are the match rates of some of the most common specialties.

PGY-1 Residency Position	M.D. Applicant Match (%)	D.O. Applicant Match (%)
Anesthesiology	70.1%	52.2%
Dermatology	11.6%	13.5%
Emergency Medicine	62.1%	77.3%
Family Medicine	87.4%	75.3%
Internal Medicine	85.4%	77.4%
Neurological Surgery	73.6%	42.9%
Neurology	63.7%	68.2%
Obstetrics-Gynecology	84.2%	67.0%
Otolaryngology	68.2%	43.2%
Orthopedic Surgery	74.8%	62.2%
Interventional Radiology	18.5%	11.5%
Pediatrics	88.8%	81.0%
Psychiatry	85.2%	68.6%
Plastic Surgery	69.9%	10.0%
Radiation Oncology	7.9%	0.0%
General Surgery	73.2%	62.1%
Thoracic Surgery	48.3%	16.7%
Vascular Surgery	69.1%	23.1%

Keep in mind that the data above are only percentages. For example, the D.O. match rate for dermatology was technically higher than the M.D. applicants. While this may be true, there were substantially more M.D. applicants getting into dermatology. Of the accepted dermatology residents, M.D. applicants made up 83.3% of all the filled positions.

You may be wondering, why are M.D. graduates considered with higher regard, despite the exact same medical education? Some of this sentiment originated from the reputation that D.O. applicants were less qualified than M.D. applicants due to lower enrollment standards. The irony, of which we have come to find, is that high medical school statistics do not exactly equate to quality physicians. Holistic, culturally diverse, and empathetic applicants with academic talent are what creates a good doctor. In my opinion, the medical education a student obtains has little reflection on the qualifications they express for a residency. At one point during my application cycle, I was going to be an osteopathic medical student. It was my only acceptance at the time, but It didn't matter, because from that point forward, I was going to be a doctor. If I hadn't been plucked away by my local M.D. state school, I would be an osteopathic medical student today. I have worked alongside many D.O. physicians and they are equally qualified if not better than their M.D. counterparts.

- **Resource**: 2021 Residency Match Data
  https://mk0nrmp3oyqui6wqfm.kinstacdn.com/wp-content/uploads/2021/05/MRM-Results_and-Data_2021.pdf

#2: Medical School Boards. A major step forward for D.O. programs was in 2020 when a merger of allopathic and osteopathic accreditation programs occurred. This resulted in ACGME-accredited residencies to recognize the COMLEX (Osteopathic medical school boards) as an equal to USMLE (allopathic medical school boards). These board scores are a necessary component to the residency match. Traditionally, M.D. applicants had to only take the USMLE, while D.O applicants had to take both USMLE and COMLEX. This is great news for osteopathic physician recognition, but it is still too early to see if the new practices will take hold at individual residency programs. While they may formally recognize the equivalency of a COMLEX score, they have far more expertise in interpreting USMLE scores. So, at this given point and time, it is still in a D.O. student's best interest to prepare for both board exams – yet another limitation these future physicians face.

#3: Salary Differences, Fact or Fiction? During your research, you may have come across some articles discussing lower salaries for osteopathic physicians. While the headline by scream "avoid osteopathic education," closer analysis will show that the findings are secondary to statistical manipulation. It is true that on average, M.D. physicians earn more than D.O. physicians based on flat salary data. What these findings neglect to highlight is that there are far more M.D. physicians in higher paying specialties. Additionally, there is a higher percentage of M.D. physicians in urban environments which can lead to artificially higher wages due to higher cost of living. **When these factors are considered, M.D. and D.O. physicians make comparable salaries.** The rate of specialization is the true indicator of potential income, although location and years' experience are other contributing factors.

If you plan on applying to osteopathic medical schools, it is important that you consider the limitations discussed above. If you find yourself holding an acceptance to both a D.O. and M.D. school, I advise you to consider the M.D. pathway. Unless there are extenuating circumstances such as exorbitant financial downsides, or considerable distance from family, it would be wise to use the M.D. advantage to your benefit. While I do not personally agree with the residency bias or stigma surrounding the D.O. degree, your goal should be to match into the residency of your dreams. By choosing to go M.D. you may have a slight edge against D.O. applicants when it comes time to match. This is particularly true for prestigious residency programs and highly specialized fields such as neurosurgery. This medical field is dramatically changing and by the time you are in the position to match this entire bias may be absolved.

Disclaimer: The limitations I have discussed are not reflective of any viewpoint that I hold and are a shared collection of information based on residency match numbers and professional sentiment.

SHOULD YOU APPLY TO D.O. SCHOOLS:

Deciding to apply to D.O. schools can be a difficult decision to make and is highly dependent on your M.D. school list or personal medical school statistics. You will have to weigh these principles against the added cost burden along with navigating a different application portal. The American Association of Colleges of Osteopathic Medicine Application Service (**AACOMAS**) must be utilized to apply to any osteopathic medical school. While there are similarities to AMCAS, there are also several unique distinctions that can that can slow down the application process. Unfortunately, you cannot "copy-and-paste" your primary application into the AACOMAS portal. While it may not take as long as filling out AMCAS, it will still be a time-consuming process. Here are some reasons you may want to apply to Osteopathic medical schools.

#1: Your medical school statistics. In general, if you are an extremely qualified applicant, it would be in your best interest to avoid applying to D.O. programs. They will likely utilize a yield-protection strategy and consider your application a healthy donation to the cause. If you are rocking a 520 MCAT, 3.90 sGPA, and unique extracurriculars, you have a relatively high probability of getting accepted to most M.D. programs. Save the time and money and focus your efforts on AMCAS, or interview preparation. If you are a borderline applicant, have an institutional action, weak extracurriculars or all the above, it would be in your best interest to apply to D.O. medical schools (perhaps even exclusively). Applicants with weaker medical school statistics but strong extracurriculars will also benefit from applying. Most osteopathic programs value holistic applicants over pure academics. For perspective, the average MCAT and GPA for allopathic medical students is 511.5 and 3.73, respectively. On the other hand, the average MCAT and GPA for osteopathic medical school students is 503.8 and 3.54. These figures alone suggest that M.D. applicants must achieve a higher academic level to secure a program admission.

#2: Your medical school list. Depending on how many medical schools you plan to apply to and the current distribution of safety, target, and reach schools, you may be inclined to add a few osteopathic programs to the list. Secondary to your lower statistics, you may find that your distribution is very top heavy with plenty of reach programs and only 1-2 safety schools. To protect yourself from the possibility of repeating the cycle, you should consider applying to D.O. schools. It will be far better to become a D.O. than it will be to face the application cycle again, which also offers no guarantees of success.

#3: Overestimation of Qualifications. While you may not want to hear this, almost every applicant overestimates how successful their application cycle will be. This can be particularly true for non-traditional pharmacy applicants like yourself. The majority of this book has been touting how "unique and special" your background is. While true in a sense, I don't want to give you any false confidence thinking your application is bullet-proof. Right now, you are operating in a vacuum and likely don't realize how many other qualified and prepared students are entering the same application cycle. Even if starting a new D.O. application can be a monstrous task, it will be worth it in the end if you can avoid re-applying. In all seriousness, once you start a pharmacy job during your gap year and see that 6-figure income, it will be very difficult to resort back to retaking the MCAT and padding your resume.

Deciding to apply early also has the same benefits seen with allopathic medical schools. It would be in your best interest to apply to AACOMAS at the same time as your AMCAS or shortly after. In mid-October, early November, there is always a large influx of osteopathic applications. This is in part due to allopathic applicants with zero interviews panicking at the realization that they may not have been as competitive as they once thought. These applicants must scramble to fill out AACOMAS prior to individual school deadlines, in the hopes of getting into a singular medical school. By applying early, you can avoid the hustle and bustle and secure an osteopathic acceptance early in the cycle. Like I already mentioned, I had an osteopathic acceptance by early November. As you know my circumstances changed, otherwise this book would be called "Pharm.D. to D.O." Don't overestimate your qualifications and add a safety net of osteopathic medical schools.

MAKING YOUR D.O. SCHOOL LIST:

To begin, you will need to sign up for the **Choose DO Explorer**. Like the MSAR, this will have application information for all 37 accredited colleges of osteopathic medicine in the United States. Similar to AMCAS, when making your school list you should pay close attention to each program's unique requirements. I want to point out that some programs have different prerequisite requirements while others request osteopathic physician letters of recommendation. While it may be fruitful for you to attempt to fulfill these requirements, your time will be better served researching the next program.

While researching you will come to find that osteopathic medical schools are extremely particular about their medical mission. While they may have lower admission statistics, they make up for it with a higher appreciation for holistic candidates. You will want to research each school's mission to find out what they are passionate about. Most will have a strong interest in primary care, community health, and rural medicine. If those characteristics are of genuine interest to you, you stand a pretty good shot at getting an interview invite. When submitting your secondary applications to osteopathic programs (yes, there are D.O. secondaries too), shift your focus to fall in line with each school's mission. While this may be a useful technique for M.D. schools, it is essential for D.O. schools.

Since you plan on applying to osteopathic programs, I recommend you apply to some of the best or most popular D.O. schools. Many of these programs have a strong reputation of producing qualified osteopathic physicians that residency programs are warming up to. It will serve you best to apply to these well-known programs because of their strong track record and promising graduate match data. The osteopathic schools below were included in U.S. News's list of top medical schools. The list is no particular order and each school falls within the rankings of 93-123. For more information about these particular programs you can visit **Shemmassian Consulting** or the Choose DO Explorer program.

1	Lake Erie College of Osteopathic Medicine (LECOM)
2	Edward Via College of Osteopathic Medicine (EVCOM)
3	Nova Southeastern University Dr. Kiran C. Patel College of Osteopathic Medicine
4	Touro University California College of Osteopathic Medicine
5	Western University of Health Sciences College of Osteopathic Medicine
6	University of North Texas Health Science Center at Fort Worth College of Osteopathic Medicine
7	Rowan University School of Osteopathic Medicine
8	Ohio University Heritage College of Osteopathic Medicine
9	University of New England College of Osteopathic Medicine
10	West Virginia School of Osteopathic Medicine
11	Lincoln Memorial University DeBusk College of Osteopathic Medicine
12	University of Pikeville – Kentucky College of Osteopathic Medicine
13	William Carey University College of Osteopathic Medicine

- **Resource**: Choose DO Explorer
  https://choosedo.org/

- **Resource**: Shemmassian Consulting Best DO Schools
  https://www.shemmassianconsulting.com/blog/best-do-schools#osteopathic-medical-school-admissions-strategies

AACOMAS: OSTEOPATHIC MEDICINE APPLICATION SERVICE:

While I am not going to cover AACOMAS with the same level of detail as I did with AMCAS, I do want to point out several key distinctions between the two application platforms. Before we dive in, review the chart below to understand the basic differences.

Area of Difference	AMCAS	AACOMAS
Personal Statement	Rationale for becoming a physician	Rationale for becoming an "osteopathic" physician
Work/Activities	700-character limit	600-character limit
	Maximum of 15 entries	No maximum
	3 most-meaningful experiences	Not applicable
	No individual achievements section	New classification for "Achievements"
Costs	$170 for the 1st school, and $42 for each additional school	$197 for the 1st school, and $48 for each additional school
Test Scores	MCAT score report will automatically populate	MCAT score report MUST be manually submitted
Number of Schools	154	37

#1: **Personal Statement**. While you may be tempted to copy and paste your personal statement from AMCAS, you may want to make some minor adjustments. Instead of describing how you want to become a physician, you will need to specifically articulate why you want to be an "osteopathic" physician.

#2: **Work/Activities.** The big distinction found here is the character count limitations. This can be one of the most frustrating parts about the entire process. You will have to adjust your pre-written AMCAS reflections to meet the lower character amount limitations. This can be challenging because I used every extra character AMCAS gave me to articulate my experiences. Throwing away a perfectly written response was painful, even if it was only a couple sentences. AACOMAS also allows applicants to report "Achievements." These are different from your traditional experiences and include any university honors (Deans List, Scholarships, Awards, etc.).

#3: **Sending MCAT Scores.** While AMCAS can automatically pull this data into your application, AACOMAS will need you to manually submit your score reports. I personally had an issue with this component because I had manually typed my MCAT scores in but forgot to submit verification score reports. There are instructions online that can help you with the transfer process.

#4: **Adding Schools is Burdensome.** Most osteopathic medical schools will have their own specific prerequisite requirements. In order to meet these requirements, you will have to designate what courses will count towards their requirements. For example, if I plan on applying to LECOM, I will need to designate in AACOMAS which courses I want to count towards LECOM's "Biology" prerequisite. This will require you to manually select from a list of all your inputted transcripts to match each class to the requirement. This is not a challenging task but can take some time if you plan on applying to multiple osteopathic programs. One benefit of doing this is that it protects you from applying to a program if you don't have the necessary prerequisites. If I lacked biochemistry credits, AACOMAS would not let me apply to a school that had the course in its requirements. This is very different from AMCAS who's hand-off approach can lead to financial loss if you aren't careful.

#5: Letters of Recommendation. As a final reminder, get an osteopathic physician letter of recommendation. It will fulfill some schools' requirements and help you support your claim that you want to be an osteopathic physician. Having shadowed one allows you to validate said claim. If you utilized the third-party letter service, Interfolio, you can easily transfer your protected letters of recommendation into AACOMAS.

- **Resource**: Interfolio Letter Delivery
  https://support.interfolio.com/m/62586/l/646844-how-to-use-dossier-deliver-for-a-medical-or-dental-school-application

PHARM.D. TO M.D.

PART EIGHT:

THE INTERVIEW

"I told my doctor I broke my leg in two places. They told me to stop going to those places."

– Henny Youngman

    How surreal is it that you are on the brink of getting into medical school? If you are reading this section, you are either impatient, curious, or have successfully been invited to an interview! It's an incredible feeling to see an interview invitation in your inbox, but ironic how quickly that excitement fades – especially when you come to the realization that YOU, yeah you, have to interview for a select few admission seats in a medical school. Potentially your dream school! The stakes are high, your career ambitions on the line, and you are surrounded by equally qualified applicants all fighting for the same thing! This is not to scare you, or provoke any anxiety, but it is a major component in the application cycle. Now that you have secured one of the few interview invites, your academics are no longer the most important factor for your application. On interview day, the admission's committee wants to see who you are as a person, how you interact with others, and determine if you are a good fit for their program.

At first interviewing can be intimidating, but the preparation is far simpler than anything you have completed leading up to it. **Additionally, the odds of getting into medical school have shifted dramatically in your favor!** Your competition went from several thousand other applicants to sometimes less than 400 other interviewees. Once you receive an interview you have approximately a 33%-50% of getting an acceptance. Far better odds than the 1-3% pre-interview probability statistics. This is certainly an achievement that should not go unnoticed. Medical schools will only interview applicants that they believe will make a positive contribution to their program. You have passed the hardest test, and just need to finish up strong. The interview will be the final touches to demonstrate that you are more than stellar on a piece of paper. They are looking for the human qualities that make for good physicians.

As we progress through this section, we will introduce a variety of different interview types, address strategies to excel, and cover some of the most common questions you should expect to receive along the way.

THE INTERVIEW TIMELINE

The process typically follows this generic schedule. You are invited for an interview and are asked to schedule your interview date. They will typically give you a few days to select between, within a month or so of time. Other medical schools will tell you the exact date and time that they want you to interview. If you have prior commitments that are unavoidable (APPE Rotations), you may need to address that specifically with the admissions office. You arrive on interview day, and will be interviewed by several faculty, usually given a tour, and several presentations about the program itself. At the conclusion of your interview day, your work is complete unless you intend to send a thank you letter. Behind the scenes, your interviewers will formally present your application file to the admission's committee with their opinions about the interview. There are three potential fates that you could face; the first is an outright acceptance, the second is being put on a waitlist, and the third is an outright rejection. If you receive an outright rejection, it's pretty safe to say you bombed the interview. While that can be disheartening, it can be an excellent wake-up call for you to work on your interview technique.

THE PHARMACY ADVANTAGE:

As pharmacy students, you have a stronger interview baseline than most of your fellow applicants. This is not to say you will pass with flying colors, but professional school tends to create professional and mature students. Pharmacy school is no exception to this rule. You will likely have more life-experience, extra years of research, far more patient encounters, and a true understanding of the rigors of graduate level education. These are qualities that cannot be taught – they fostered through personal growth and achievement. If you are a pharmacy student reading this book, in all likelihood, you are one of the aforementioned applicants. Don't let it get to your head though. The last thing you want to do is come across as pretentious, arrogant, or dismissive. A school representative will pick-up on this and your chances of getting into the school will plummet dramatically.

Your interview starts the second you set food on campus. Everyone you encounter could be a potential informant to the admissions board. Be your best self, stay humble and do your homework on each school! I am only sharing this because you will be surprised how natural interviewing feels, especially since you have probably felt out of place throughout the entire application cycle. I personally found interview season to be the most enjoyable aspect of applying to medical school, and hopefully you will too!

DIFFERENT INTERVIEW TYPES & STRATEGIES:

Believe it or not, there is more than one way to conduct an interview, outside of the traditional one-on-one you may be familiar with. Medical schools like to employ a variety of different interview methods to investigate different characteristics that an applicant may or may not have. For example, an applicant may be a rockstar during a traditional one-on-one interview but is horrible working with others, as seen in a group-interview.

Prior to your interview day you will conduct extensive research on the types of interviews each medical school utilizes. Some medical schools stick to the classics while others create a hybrid of each specific type. Before we attempt to tackle interview preparation techniques, we need to introduce each interview style that you could come up against.

#1: The Traditional Interview. You should be familiar with this style of interviewing. It consists of a one-on-one or a panel of interviewers asking you standardized questions. The allotted time ranges anywhere from 15 minutes to 1 hour. Your interviewer is typically a member of the admissions committee but could also be a faculty member, community leader, current student, or affiliate clinician. The style of your discussion is usually casual, starting with a few standard questions that will slowly transition into a general conversation. The interviewer wants to get a sense of who you are as a person and see if you are sociable. Keep in mind that each interviewer will be different and have their own methods for interviewing a student. Therefore, it is difficult to predict how your interview will play out.

Your interview can either be an open or closed book format. Meaning that your interviewer may or may not have access to your submitted material. A closed interview is utilized to eliminate bias based on your medical school statistics. Your entire conversation and everything you choose to reveal will be new to your interviewer. If that is the case, you should do your best to highlight some of the key facets about your application, including your unique educational background. I have had interviewers who were fascinated with my pharmacy background, and we talked about medicine, medications, and patient care for the entire interview! I felt more like a colleague instead of a poor applicant begging for a seat at the medical school table. I anticipate you will have similar experiences, especially during your longer interviews.

#2: The Group-Interview. This is exactly as it sounds. You will be packed into a room with several other applicants sometimes as many as 10 others. These interviews are designed to see how well applicants can work in a group setting and highlight interpersonal shortcomings. These shortcomings include controlling attitudes, arrogant or dismissive behavior, and major social awkwardness. These qualities are not conducive to becoming a good physician and medical schools want to pick-up on this before they offer you one of the coveted seats in their program. During the group interview you should expect to work alongside your fellow students. You may be given a variety of different questions including some of the ones discussed below, or various ethical scenarios. When the session begins make sure you don't talk over your fellow peers or hijack the entire room when making your points. You should aim to talk several times and contribute different perspectives but acknowledge the previous speakers' points.

- **Introduce yourself when the session starts.** Don't jump the gun too soon as the session instructor will likely ask everyone to share a little about themselves. During this part, make sure you pay attention to everyone's name. Also try to keep your introduction short. No one likes that applicant who feels like they need share their life story instead of sticking to the "fun fact question." If you don't understand this quite yet, you will on interview day!

- **Listen carefully when others speak.** Avoid repeating content that has already been discussed unless you feel as though it was left incomplete. Paying attention can also allow you to add to a previous applicant's comment, strengthening an argument. Do not let your mind wander, especially when other applicants may directly ask you a question. This is absolutely critical.

- **Be aware of your body language.** You may have no interest at all in the topic discussed or your fellow applicant is holding everyone hostage with their 5-minute introduction. Be patient and act as if whoever is talking is the most important person in the room. Poor body language although subtle can make you look disinterested or dismissive. These are qualities that can lead to a quick rejection.

- **Take charge or become the group discussion leader.** Although this is not always necessary or may not be appropriate for the task at hand, it can be a great way to demonstrate your leadership skills. Survey the room and pay attention to see if your fellow applicants are gravitating to you or are agreeing with your points. Informally become the group leader. This isn't about outshining your peers, but rather a necessary step in creating a strong functioning team to accomplish the task at hand. This would be a great opportunity to show that you can handle groupwork and can read the room. If another individual is slowly taking on the role, acknowledge their efforts and you could appoint them yourself. Recognizing other talents in the room can demonstrate humility and awareness for what may be best for the group. Moderators will pick up on these tiny details, which can contribute to a successful interview.

- **Make sure everyone's voice is heard**. You don't want to be the student who over-dominates the discussion and shuts out others. This is a pathologic strategy that many applicants fall victim to. You need to encourage healthy discussion amongst your peers and get others involved. Some students may feel overwhelmed or shy and won't speak unless spoken to. Ask them what they think about the current point of discussion or to share their thoughts with the group.

- **Don't be afraid to disagree.** Alternatively, it would be unwise to challenge another group member's ideas with a hostile tone. You are entitled to your opinion, but make sure your approach is constructive. At points during your group interview, some applicants may suggest ideas that are not the best for the group. It's okay to provide a little push back and you may notice that other students will come to support you. You could easily suggest an improvement of the idea rather than completely reshaping the concept at hand. The Admissions Board wants to see if you can effectively resolve conflict while making sure you maintain your composure.

#3: Multiple Mini-Interviews (MMIs). The name says it all! The format consists of 5-10 interview stations. At each station you will have a prompt/short paragraph to read outside each office door. You are given approximately 2 minutes to read the prompt and collect your thoughts. After the reading period ends, you will enter the room and talk about the prompt and/or answer any questions from an interviewer sitting in the room. These individual stations are short, and students only have 5-8 minutes for discussion. These interviews are typically closed file, and the interviewer will have no access to any of your records. Their primary purpose is to assess your critical thinking skills and ethical decision making. While these same principles are investigated during a traditional and group interview, the MMIs provide more reliable data. This is particularly true due to the higher number of evaluators who can grade you compared to 1-2 people in a traditional interview setting.

Preparing for MMIs can be challenging because it is very hard to predict what questions you may come across. You could theoretically review hundreds of potential questions and practice your responses with others, but your best bet will be to check out Student Doctor Network's university specific questions (more information about this in the next section). I have listed some potential scenarios you could come across below!

1. An interaction with an actor or the medical school's standardized patient.

2. A traditional interview station.

3. A teamwork station where you are paired with another student and must solve a problem at hand.

4. An ethical station asking you to discuss social or policy-based problems.

5. A personal essay station (sometimes given double the time).

INTERVIEW PREPARATION:

Interview preparation is very straight-forward and gets easier the more interviews you complete. At first you may spend an entire week preparing for your interviews and hardly sleeping throughout. You'll find yourself creating a google document, writing out responses to every potential question, and researching a program's mission statement until you can recite it from memory. While completing these tasks are necessary to have a successful interview, by the time you reach your last interview, you will be surprised how little preparation you will need. If I had $1 for every time I had rehearsed the "why not pharmacy" question in my head, I could probably retire right now. I hope you will find this news encouraging and enjoy preparing for interviews!

#1: Create a Student Doctor Network (SDN) account. This is a phenomenal platform that should be used throughout the application cycle to find answers to common questions. I used it frequently to supplement material from reddit during my application cycle. The most important aspect concerning this website isn't the various subtopic discussions, but a comprehensive list of medical school interview questions. Not only do they have a massive list of questions, but they are specific for each medical school. What more could you possibly ask for?

For example, let us say you received an interview invite from Loyola University Stritch School of Medicine. By navigating through Student Doctor Network's website, you will be able to see the various questions that previous applicants had on their interview day. The questions are subdivided into various sections including 1st, 2nd, 3rd questions received, most interesting question, most difficult question, and so on. Each medical school has the option to change their interview questions each cycle but generally refrain from doing so. Use this Student Doctor Network resource! To find the interview questions, follow the steps below.

1. Go to the home page.

2. Hover your mouse over the "Resources" dropdown.

3. Select "MD Applicants."

4. This will bring you to a new page, again hover your mouse over the "Resources" dropdown.

5. Click on "Interview Feedback."

6. Search your school of interest.

If this material isn't enough for you, you can also check out the 500 Interview Question document referenced previously.

#2: Read each medical school's website. Prior to your interview you will need to become an expert on the respective medical school. You will need to be familiar with the school mission, research opportunities, community service clubs, recent changes in the curriculum, and opportunities for medical students to get involved. This is like the secondary essay prompt "why us?" but on steroids. For your interview day, you should be that medical school's personal expert.

#3: Know your application in and out. Anything you have ever sent to this particular medical school (including AMCAS and Secondary Applications) is fair game during the interview. I have been on interviews where they had my application printed and the interviewer pointed out different things asking for clarification. It could happen to you so be ready to defend or expand any content that you provided. If you have an institutional action, be prepared for the inevitable follow-up questions. They will ask. You have been warned!

#4: Practice with someone else. Have your partner/family/friend ask you various questions in a mock-interview format. Having another individual judging your responses can help you formulate better answers and add some healthy pressure. Ask your practice buddy for feedback on social performance as well. Did you make good eye-contact, maintain your posture, avoid fidgeting? These important social queues can detract from even the strongest question answers. Lastly, don't over-practice. By over practicing you are at risk for perfectly memorizing your answers. This can result in your responses coming across as robotic and cold, a huge negative when your primary purpose is to demonstrate the human qualities you hold.

#5: Prepare to ask your own questions. This is just as much of an interview for the medical school as it is for your you. If a particular school presents itself in a manner that you feel would not fit your personality, take note of this. Do the current students look miserable and tired, or complain about the lack of comradery amongst their peers? These are important queues to pick up on. The last thing you need is to commit to a medical school that will make you miserable, especially if you have other acceptances. If at the end of the day it's your only acceptance, you'll have to remain steadfast and push through.

Asking questions is also an important technique that advances your understanding of a program and demonstrates to the admissions board that you are interested in what they have to offer. While asking questions on your campus tour can help you stand-out in the crowd, you don't want to come off as too eager or obnoxious. I've seen it many times how 1 or 2 applicants on interview day become the tour guide's shadow. Don't be that person! If you are going to ask a lot of questions, make sure its during your interviews, primarily if it is a traditional interview.

Here is a list of questions you should consider asking on interview day. This list is far from comprehensive. Also, try to reserve these for your traditional interview time slots. Asking questions can help fill an awkward silence while showing that you are engaged.

1. Why did you choose to teach?

2. Why did you choose your particular specialty?

3. What important experiences/events have led you to the position you are in today?

4. What is your favorite book? Do you have any recommendations on what I should read?

5. What do you look for in a medical student?

6. What are some of your favorite things to do in this city/town?

7. What is your typical day like as a physician/faculty?

8. What clubs/programs do you think benefit current students the most?

9. How would you describe the student faculty relationship at this medical school?

10. Could you tell me more about the curriculum, and organization of courses?

11. What are you most excited about concerning the future of medicine?

QUESTIONS TO EXPECT:

As a pharmacy student there are several questions you should expect to receive throughout your interview season. While the questions themselves are intuitive, its highly important that you have a strong answer. As someone with a unique background and a crazy desire to switch out of an already successful profession, you will need to justify doing so. Take a look at these important questions and brainstorm your own ideas!

#1: *"Why medicine? Why not pharmacy?"*

This is the #1 most common question I received during interviews. Your fellow interviewees will ask, the current medical students at the program will ask, heck even the barista at the hospital coffee shop will want to know what you are doing here. Brainstorm a positive way to praise pharmacy while also accepting that you wanted more, or to do more with your degree. I tackled this question by telling a story. "I started pharmacy because of "X." As I progressed through school and learned about pathology I was fascinated with medicine. I shadowed Dr. "Y" which solidified my desire to pursue medicine. I want to work directly with patients, develop personal relationships, and direct care using my pharmaceutical knowledge and newfound perspective." Input your own experiences into this example, or better yet, create a far more insightful rationale than this one!

#2: *"What have you been doing in your gap-year?"*

This question is a common secondary prompt, but some programs like to ask it in interviews too. Their purpose is to see if you have been productive leading up to a potential medical school matriculation, especially since it has likely been months since your last point of contact via application submissions. To answer this question, think of your APPE rotation experiences. Most interviewers will have no idea how involved a pharmacy student can be on clinical rounds. Your responsibilities are similar to a medical student's. You work up patients, present information to the team, and make medication recommendations to improve patient care. My preceptor would often send me on medical rounds alone and I would serve as the acting pharmacist for periods of time. I am sure you have similar experiences of independence. These are critical events that you should communicate to your interviewer, to demonstrate that you are already a qualified healthcare professional.

#3: *"Issues within healthcare"*

These include any medically related hot-topics. Your interviewer wants to see if you are an informed and interested in medicine, outside of padding your own resume. Prior to any interview, you should research various topics that have the potential to come up in discussion. Your entire angle for the interview focuses on how "intelligent, and involved you are as a pharmacy student." Prove it by demonstrating your personal knowledge on these topics.

As a pharmacy student, you should already have a baseline understanding of some of these issues through your education, work experiences, or clinical rotations. As a healthcare professional, you have the opportunity to knock these questions out of the park. Alternatively, your fellow competing applicants have likely only reviewed the Wikipedia page the night prior. Important topics that you should investigate include, the opioid epidemic, naloxone utilization, the anti-vaxxer movement, American healthcare issues, cost of medications and so on! Keep in mind that there is usually no correct answer so take a side but respectfully accept that others are entitled to different viewpoints.

#4: *"Why do you want to attend our program?"*

Also, a similar question seen on secondary applications. Most medical schools want to reiterate this point and extract more information from you. They want to ensure that you really are as passionate about their program as you claim to be. One of the biggest mistakes students make answering this question is that they talk about the amenities the institution has to offer, particularly what they like about the school. While this does demonstrate that you either did your homework, or paid attention on the tour, it lacks the rationale for why you belong in their program. To correctly approach this question, you need to articulate why you are a great fit for these specific programs, and how they will benefit from having you.

For example, a bad answer would be *"this medical school has a world class hospital, and cutting edge curriculum that facilitated the development of qualified physicians."* While these points may ring true, you have only listed known facts.

Instead, you should reply, *"One of the biggest reasons I'm drawn to school [XYZ] is because of its strong academic medical center and affiliate hospital. Students have access to clinical resources and physician shadowing right from the get-go which allows students to apply their textbook knowledge to real life clinical scenarios. Doing so during the first few months of medical school puts everything into perspective and helps learners appreciate why we do what we do. As a pharmacist, I believe that my clinical experiences would be a great asset to my fellow peers by helping with medication questions and fostering patient-centered decision-making skills."*

#5: *"What is your biggest weakness?"* or *"Tell me a time you failed."*

This question often gives students plenty of trouble. It can be difficult to think of a limitation to your application especially when all you have done the last few months is talk about how great you are. This question is a great opportunity to display self-awareness and that you can be introspective. Interviewers want to see if you can acknowledge a shortcoming, and then overcome this limitation for the better. Please do not attempt to use a fake weakness, such as being a "perfectionist," or you "work too hard." An interviewer will see right through this and your chances of getting accepted will be diminished.

The basic formula to tackle this question is as follows. Discuss a weakness or failure that you demonstrated in an experience. Talk about how it impacted you, or others, and that you recognized it may not have been the most appropriate/thoughtful way to act. Shift your direction by addressing how you corrected the misgiving and what you learned from the event. Finally reflect on the overall experience and discuss how you will apply your new perspective to act better in your future endeavors.

THANK YOU LETTERS:

Now that you have finished your interview, you have one final task. This section is completely optional, but the gesture is always appreciated. Thank you letters demonstrate professionalism and show your interviewer that you valued their time. Be aware that each medical school will have different expectations for thank you letters. Some programs will have built-in locations on your application portal to upload a letter, while other programs will have you directly contact your interviewer. Remember, at least one of your interviewers will be reporting your application to the admissions board. If they were previously on the fence about your interview, a kind letter may shift their disposition to your favor. While most interviewers would deny that the formality had any influence, you never know what goes on behind the scenes.

Also, most interviewers will work with several other applicants during the long day. Seeing so many different qualified students in one day can make you blend in with the others. Sending a letter can make you stand-out of the crowd and remind them just how great you were. When writing your letter, discuss a memorable point of conversation you had during the interview. For example, I remembered discussing book recommendations with my interviewer, so I was sure to follow-up in my thank you letter with the very same point. Take a look at my example thank you email to the admission's coordinator and the interviewer specific thank you letter.

NATHAN M. GARTLAND

Email Content:

Hi Mrs. Smith,

I hope you are enjoying your weekend! Thank you for the wonderful interview experience on Saturday, February 1st. I appreciated the inclusive and friendly environment portrayed by The School of Medicine's faculty and student representatives. Everyone at the interview was very welcoming and emphasized the collaborative nature of program. I was very impressed and would be honored to be admitted to the [XYZ] School of Medicine.

Additionally, I have attached my two-interviewer specific thank you letters in this email. I was unsure if I should send them to you, or directly to Dr. [Rachels] and Dr. [Brighton]. I would appreciate it if you would be able to forward these letters to my interviewers or provide me with their email addresses/mailing addresses if necessary. My AMCAS number is 12345678 for your reference. Please let me know what I can do to ensure that the letters are received.

Thank you for your help and the warm introduction to [XYZ] University!

Sincerely,

Nathan M. Gartland

PHARM.D. TO M.D.

Interviewer Specific Thank You:

[*Your Name*]
[*Email Address*]
[*Your Street Address*]
[*Your City, State, Zip code*]
[*Phone Number*]

[*Todays Date*]

[*Charles M. Brighton*], M.D.
[*XYZ*] School of Medicine
Department of Family Medicine

Dear Dr. [*Brighton*],

Thank you so much for taking time out of your busy schedule to interview me for a position in the [*XYZ*] School of Medicine on February 1st. I thoroughly enjoyed our conversation during our brief meeting and appreciated your thoughtful inquiry into my pharmacy background. I especially enjoyed the relaxed nature of the interview and the friendly environment embodied by the School of Medicine faculty. It was pleasant to discuss the intricacies of the opioid crisis, your personal contributions to underserved populations, as well as some financial books such as *Loonshots*. I found your commitment to patient care to be inspiring and reflective of a [*XYZ*] medical education.

Throughout the interview day, the staff and current medical students exhibited a passionate zeal for the program and emphasized the collaborative mentality of their peers. Everyone I spoke with was very accepting and excited to share their personal experiences of the program. The sense of family and commitment to others has genuinely strengthened my desire to receive a medical education at [*XYZ*].

Additionally, I found the School of Medicine's state of the art facilities and educational technology to be very impressive, and reflective of the university's passion for a quality medical education. I was thrilled to learn about the remodelled course curriculum as well as the opportunity for patient interaction within the first professional year. The School of Medicine's presence in the community is unmatched and represents a culture truly dedicated to the service of underserved populations. I look forward to utilizing my pharmacy training to further academic, professional, and patient centered endeavours at this respected school of medicine. I am hopeful that the Admissions Committee will consider me to be worthy of acceptance into the medical family at [*XYZ*].

Thank you again for the wonderful opportunity to share my experiences and learn more about the [*XYZ*] School of Medicine.

Sincerely,

    Insert Signature Here

TAKEAWAYS:

- Now that you have an interview, the odds of getting an acceptance have shifted in your favor.

- As a pharmacy student you will have a professional advantage when it comes to interview skills.

- Medical schools commonly employ a variety of interview subtypes including the traditional one-on-one, the group interview, and MMIs.

- Research the school you are interviewing at and look-up previous interview questions from The Student Doctor Network.

- Expect the obvious questions and have strong answers.

- Send thank you letters even if the program declares that doing so will not impact your chances. It never hurts to be a professional!

PHARM.D. TO M.D.

PART NINE:

THE PRE/POST-INTERVIEW LIMBO

"If opportunity doesn't knock, build a door."

– Milton Berle

You have been through it all at this point. You have finished all your applications, attended several interviews or are still waiting, all while completing your APPE rotations. Regardless, your cycle is almost complete. This section will address minor details concerning the stretch of time between secondary submissions and the final day of the application cycle.

For those of you who are still waiting for interview invites, be patient. Please do not base the success of your cycle off other applicants boasting online. You will see people in the reddit and student doctor network forums celebrating interviews and acceptances but don't let that get in your head! After you submit your last secondary, you may go six months without a single communication. You may also get five interviews in the first week. Every single person will have a slightly different experience so don't get tangled up in all the chatter. All it takes is one interview and one acceptance. It's very easy to get caught up in the cycle so don't forget to have fun along the way!

UNDERSTANDING WAITLISTS:

You are probably familiar with the variety of potential status changes your application may experience during the cycle. As the cycle rolls out medical schools will begin to group the massive number of applications they receive. Some of these classifications include the pre-interview waitlist, offering an interview invite, or an outright rejection. Following the interview applicants can then be processed and placed on a post-interview waitlist, receive an outright acceptance or receive an outright rejection. This section is designed to give you a better understanding of waitlists and what to expect when placed on each particular type. **Unfortunately, it is near impossible to predict how quickly students will be moved from the waitlist.** The number varies with every cycle and is dependent on the number of interview or acceptance withdrawals that a particular medical school has. Some medical schools have approximately 33% of their current class coming off the waitlist, while others have less than 2%. Getting put on a waitlist can be a scary, and disappointing reality that many applicants face. I was placed on several post-interview waitlists, one of which I got off, while the others I withdrew from.

#1: Pre-interview waitlist. This is never a good sign. Most medical schools only offer several hundred interviews every cycle. In order to ensure that those interview slots get filled, they place students on a waitlist who they can call upon in case one of the actual interview slot holders withdraws. Interview withdrawals are usually uncommon, especially early in the cycle. The only reasons a student would withdrawal from an interview is that they are already holding an acceptance, or they no longer wished to attend a program. Students on this waitlist can expect to wait extremely long times before getting the final decision. Most online blogs and forums consider this a "Soft Rejection." While this can be disappointing, students get off these lists every, so in the end it is still better than an outright rejection!

#2: Post-interview Waitlist. You finished the interview but didn't exactly wow the admissions board. You find yourself on a post-interview waitlist which is less than ideal. You are thinking to yourself, where did I go wrong? Please don't torture yourself. Depending on how early you interviewed you have a reasonable chance of moving off the list. Research the current program's waitlist policies and gather insight from previous/current applicants to see how quickly the waitlist moves. I doubt you will find any direct or official answers but some of the online responses can give you peace of mind. The movement of the waitlist is highly specific to each medical school so you will have to adjust your expectations accordingly.

Additionally, some medical schools utilize a "rank list" associated with their waiting list. Essentially, applicants who interviewed are ranked on their performance during interview day. They are assigned a hidden score by the medical school and are placed on the post-interview waitlist. You may have been extremely qualified and could potentially be number 1 or 2 on the waitlist. You may also have performed poorly and could be so far down on the list that a kinder gesture would have been an outright rejection. There is no possible way to know how each school generates and organizes its waitlist so if you are placed on one, it's probably best to not stress about it.

PHARM.D. TO M.D.

PROVIDE UPDATE LETTERS TO PROGRAMS:

This is your opportunity to highlight any key improvements to your resume since you submitted all your application materials. This is also an excellent way to express your interest in a program and get off a pre or post-interview waitlist. If you have been following the schedule, you will have completed your secondaries by September and should now be in the waiting phase. You are at the mercy of the medical schools and their will to grant you an interview or an acceptance. However, this period is not entirely passive, and you can submit an update letter to the programs of your choosing. Do your research and find out what schools on your list accept updates and find out how they accept them. The last thing you want to do is spend time creating a personalized update letter for a program that will reject your efforts.

Make sure the content you provide in the update letter is **substantial and of the highest quality**. Recent publications, an incredible patient experience, or a respectable new position in the hospital. This is a fantastic opportunity for a pharmacy student to broadcast their unique APPE rotations and demonstrate the clinical nature of their involvement. As you will see, some rotations will have you take on minimal responsibility, while others will have you work independently. These make for unique stories that the Admissions Committee will love to hear. Your PY4 year is also the time when much of your pharmacy related research will come to fruition. As pharmacy students, many of you will have been working towards presenting your work at the American Society of Health-System Pharmacists (ASHP) Mid-year Clinical Meeting. What is normally a showcase for residency and fellowship applicants can be a great opportunity for you to present a poster or give a stand-out presentation. This is yet another excellent opportunity to demonstrate your passion for research and the propagation of medicine, and certainly a worthy addition to your update letter.

Don't send updates until you have given programs some time to process your application. You do not want to be that applicant who submits an update 20 minutes after completing the same school's secondary. They will wonder why you did not include that information on your recently submitted contents, and it may negatively impact you. Unfortunately, I cannot tell you how long that will be because everyone applies at different times, but generally November or December are reasonable times to submit. Here are a few examples of when you should consider sending an update letter.

- If you have interviewed at the program and haven't heard from them in a while.

- If you have been placed on a Pre-Interview Waitlist, a letter may remind them that you still exist and are doing great things.

- If you have had no updates about the status of your application since you finished your submission, an update letter might jolt them to look into your profile.

Lastly, even if you don't have anything substantial to update your medical schools with (unlikely with your APPE Rotations), many programs will consider your letter a sign that you are still interested in their program. It will also serve as a touchpoint opportunity where you can contact the program again and let them know that you are "extremely excited to hear from them." Sending update letters successfully moved me from at least one pre-interview waitlist. I think it was worth it!

Provided below is an example template of an update letter as well as a complete update letter that I produced and submitted during my application cycle. Feel free to use a similar style or this outline to get you started. Don't forget to individualize the content to fit your personality and experiences.

PHARM.D. TO M.D.

The Format:

Name
Email
AMCAS#
Address

Date

School Name
Office of Admissions Title
Address

Introduction Statement,

Updates:
- Completed Clinical Rotations (Including a patient centered experience)
- New case-based presentations while on rotations or conferences
- Research Advances or Relevant Publication Updates

Closing Statements (how your new experiences make you an excellent fit at their program)

    Signature (electronically signed)

    Name

Complete Example:

John Doe
Medstudent@gmail.com
AMCAS ID#: 12345678
123 S Towsen Ave.
Philadelphia, PA 12345

November 20, 2019

[XYZ] School of Medicine
Office of Admissions
987 Elmwood Avenue, Box 123A
Rochester, NY 98765

To Whom It May Concern,

    I am writing today to provide The Admissions Committee with an update of my recent activity for the 2019 fall semester. As I continue to work towards my pharmacy doctoral degree, I have completed several **new patient-centered clinical rotations** since the submission of my secondary application in July. More specifically, these experiences encompassed five weeks of full-time work at an Outpatient Anticoagulation Clinic, and Neurosurgical Intensive Care Unit at Allegheny General Hospital in Pittsburgh Pennsylvania. I have also completed a five-week rotation rounding in the Neurocritical Care Unit at the Cleveland Clinic, Main Campus, in Cleveland Ohio. During my anticoagulation clinic rotation, I had the incredible opportunity to conduct multiple patient interviews that focused on managing patient's newly prescribed warfarin medication. I worked directly with my patients on a daily basis discussing medication interventions, dosage adjustments and adverse events under professional supervision. During my tenure, I found the extensive patient interaction in a primary care setting to be very rewarding as I watched my patients recover and learn while building professional relationships. All three of these rotations have broadened my understanding of medical practice and have allowed me to grow professionally and personally through actively working alongside patients and provider teams.

Additionally, while on clinical rotations, I conducted several **formal case-based presentations** to hospital staff. More specifically, three of my presentations were titled *Ketamine Use for Refractory Status Epilepticus: A Case Review*, *Therapeutic Management of Endocarditis*, and *Acute Ischemic Stroke: Primary and Secondary Management*. These formal presentations allowed me to evaluate guideline recommendations and practice standards of care to develop educational content.

Over the past few months, my research projects have come to fruition as **I have been accepted to present two unique posters** at The American Society of Health-System Pharmacists Midyear Clinical Meeting. This conference is the largest professional pharmacy gathering in the country and will be held this December in Las Vegas, Nevada. I am excited to take my clinical research findings and present them to the medical community. I believe that my passion for medical research aligns with The University of [XYZ] School of Medicine's mission for research advancement.

Lastly, I would like to inform the admissions committee that my cancer research contributions have resulted in **authorship on the manuscript,** and it has been accepted for publication in The Journal of Cellular Biochemistry as of August 29, 2019: The publication can be found at the DOI: 10.1002/jcb.12345. The title of the publication is as follows; *The Pharmacological inhibition of the MEK5/ERK5 and PI3K/Akt signaling pathways synergistically reduces viability in triple-negative breast cancer*.

I hope this update will assist the admissions committee as they continue to review my application for a seat in The University of [XYZ] School of Medicine Class of 2024. Thank you for your time and consideration.

Sincerely,

Insert Signature Here

LETTER OF INTENT (LOI):

Are you on a post-interview Waitlist? Was the school you interviewed at the program of your dreams? Is it the only school you have heard from and really need to get in? If you said yes to any of these questions, then you should consider writing a letter of Intent (LOI). This is a document you submit that allows you express your profound interest in the specific program and make a pledge to attend said program if accepted. Sound familiar? If you were thinking of the Early Decision Program, then you would be correct. The main differences are that a LOI is less formal, and you are under no obligation to carry out your pledge. I recommend that if you choose to write one of these letters, that you uphold your pledge, but I also understand that circumstances can change at a moment's notice. LOIs are typically reserved as a last-ditch effort towards the end of the application cycle.

When writing an LOI, you should reserve doing so until after you have had your interview. Particularly if you have been placed on a post-interview waitlist. Sorry to pre-interview wait-listers and those ghosted during the cycle. The purpose of the LOI is to exclaim your fascination or commitment to a program and doing so without ever setting foot on campus can be a difficult sell. Writing your LOI after your interview decision can help move you off the waitlist. While it is difficult to say how successful this task is, it certainly can't hurt.

If you haven't interviewed yet, you technically can still send an LOI. Doing so is usually ineffective, and can come across as disingenuous, but then again, "what do you have to lose?" You can boost your chances of success if you have strong family ties to the region, a legacy advantage, or experience working with students in the program. At the end of the day, you need to do what is best for your application cycle!

If you do choose to write one of these (referring to my post-interview waitlisted friends), try to wait until the program has finished their interview cycle. Most medical schools state on their website that they will stop interviewing in early to late March. Send your letter right around this time period to show the school that you are still very interested in their program. By doing so you have conveniently reminded the admissions committee that you are still eagerly awaiting their blessing. At that point in the cycle, medical schools will begin to sift through the waitlist pile of applications. Most applicants who have received acceptances will be making final decisions and any other acceptances they hold will be sent to other qualified students on the waitlist.

I was fortunate in that I never have to write a LOI, but the format is similar to an update letter with additional "fluff." These letters can get much more personal and should resonate around why you are such a great fit for the program of interest. Your letter should not be any longer than a page. Some specific points to address in your letter are listed below.

- Express your gratitude for receiving an interview and considering your application.

- Positive qualities related to the school and how they align with your own characteristics.

- Clear and unambiguous statement expressing your intent to attend the school if admitted.

- Any accomplishments you have had since your interview, including new APPE rotations.

- How you contribute to the school's diversity and how you will be a positive influence if accepted.

- Reasons for why you love the city and community the school is located in.

When submitting your LOI, send it directly to the Dean of Admissions to ensure that your letter isn't lost. Some medical schools will have an online portal location to upload additional material so make sure you follow the medical schools' protocols. Deviating from their requests can hurt your application more than it helps.

NO FORMAL UNDERGRADUATE DEGREE:

This section is reserved for a very small subset of pharmacy-based applicants who will have medical school admission delays related to incomplete application requirements. In other words, there are some medical schools who will consider your application incomplete if you do not have a "Bachelor's Degree" on your transcript. That is correct – I had my application placed on "hold" by several medical schools because my pharmacy doctorate education did not fulfill the bachelor's degree requirements. Fortunately, this can be easily corrected with several communications with the admissions department at each university. The downside was that it took several weeks for the communication to shift my application off hold. While not a huge deal in the grand scheme of things for early applicants, late applicants can experience some frustration as your application can be delayed even further. I wanted to share this information, although rare, because it is still a real possibility!

PHARMACY REDICNECY APPLICATIONS:

When applying to medical school you may want to consider applying to pharmacy residency programs. Following through with a pharmacy residency application right after completing months of medical school applications is no easy task and borderline crazy. I applaud you if you follow through!

Most applicants who are considering this potential option are doing so to hedge their medical school bet. Consider it a contingency plan for an unsuccessful application cycle. Some pharmacy students would prefer to pursue a PGY-1 pharmacy residency than to sit around and reapply. I completely understand! Why put your life on hold when you already have the potential for an incredible pharmacy career. Completing a residency will also significantly bolster your application if you are considering reapplying in the next cycle. While this idea may seem like an appealing backup plan, there are a few considerations you should keep in mind.

#1: Don't go through the match unless you are sure you want to complete a pharmacy residency. If you are considering this process you need to be absolutely sure that you would be happy with either outcome. If you decide to attend pharmacy residency interviews you are more than welcome to, BUT do not participate in the residency match unless you are going to go through with it. If you do match it is *expected* that you commit to the program. However, it technically isn't required, unless the program itself has a legal agreement that you should look into. You may find yourself matching into a pharmacy residency thinking your medical school chances have evaporated, only to find out in June that you made it off a waitlist. Turning down a residency is not only unprofessional, but unfair to both the program and your fellow pharmacy peers who may not have matched. As you know, pharmacy is a small world and you may be "black-listed" at a hospital, or even a hospital system. I recommend that you consider a residency, only if you couldn't see yourself doing anything else. I personally wanted to go to medical school no matter what, so I was already willing to work a causal job for a year then reapply. I figured doing a residency during my off year would have been too much of a commitment when medicine was my ultimate goal. **Don't settle for something that you aren't truly passionate about.** You will need to decide for yourself if this is the right path for you.

#2: Know the timing schedule. Your medical school application cycle will be in the full swing of things by the time you will need to apply to pharmacy residency programs. You may be under the impression that your chances of getting into medical school are long gone despite it only being December or January. Keep your head up! I got the majority of my M.D. interview invites in January, and February. The cycle isn't over until it's over. Despite this advice, you may want to apply to pharmacy residencies anyway. If you are seriously considering it, you should attend the ASHP Mid-year Clinical Meeting and talk with each pharmacy residency program of interest. I am not going to tell you how to apply to pharmacy residency programs. You will likely have far better insight from your pharmacy school faculty! I just want you to be aware that it might be a little too soon to throw in the towel for your medical school applications.

#3: Added expenses: The medical school application cycle is already extremely overpriced. Applying to pharmacy programs will subtract more funds from your already strained bank account. PhORCAS (the residency application service) costs $110 for the first 4 programs, and then an additional $43 per program. This doesn't even factor in the cost of residency interview travel. This is not a cheap process so be warned!

PHARM.D. TO M.D.

PART TEN:

HOLDING A MEDICAL SCHOOL ACCEPTANCE

"You know what they call the fellow who finishes last in their medical school graduating class? They call them 'Doctor.'"

– Abe Lemons

You now hold a medical school acceptance, and if you have had a strong cycle, multiple acceptances. Congratulations the book worked! I recommend you resist putting it down to listen to a few important considerations regarding picking your future medical school.

So how do you decide what program you should go to? Well, if you have a singular acceptance, it's pretty self-explanatory. If you have multiple, it is not much harder. **Go to the cheapest medical school. That's it.** You will not regret this decision, especially down the road. The education you receive will be almost identical between different programs so select the one that will cost you the least. With that said, there are circumstances in which you may wish to reconsider this point. This would include choosing between a D.O. program and an M.D. program. If you are interested in a competitive specialty or a career in academia, choose the M.D. program, even if it's more expensive. Despite the progressive trends, you have a better opportunity matching into your desired specialty if you are an M.D. applicant. If you are comfortable matching into a non-competitive specialty and less resistant to travel, you should pick the cheaper D.O. program. Additionally, if the more expensive program is closer to home, or significantly more prestigious, you may want to consider these factors as well.

ACCEPTING YOUR ACCEPTANCE:

It may take some time before you come down from your personal high. You have finally made it. You achieved the goal of your dreams, and have worked so hard to get to this moment! While you are busy celebrating there are a few things you need to keep in mind when moving on to the next stage of your life. Consider these the final tasks to solidify your position as an incoming medical student. While accepting the offer from your medical school may sound intuitive, there are other tasks at hand to occupy you further.

#1: Designate your enrollment plans. Utilizing AMCAS's Choose Your Medical School Tool, you will need to designate if you "plan to enroll" or "commit to enroll." The earliest you can designate "plan to enroll" is February 19th for the current application cycle. This is an important step for medical school traffic regulations which allows them to track who is interested in attending their program. Staring April 30th, applicants can then designate "commit to enroll." This is the final step designating that you will attend the school selected. All other medical schools that offered you a seat will be alerted that you are essentially "off the table" and can then move applicants from waitlists to fill your once held acceptance slot.

#2: Access Financial Aid. Your future medical school will have likely shared some information regarding financial aid, but you should request further information pertaining to scholarships. Many medical schools have a large pool of scholarship money that they assign out to students who qualify or apply. This may not be commonly advertised so reaching out can open the door to financial support.

You should also handle your pharmacy school debt. Contact your loan supplier and get information on deferment periods and let them know that you will be continuing your education. Your new medical school should supply them with enrollment information, but it never hurts to double check.

PHARMACY BOARDS:

You already know how passionate I am about pharmacy so neglecting your education by disregarding licensure is rather foolish in my opinion. I understand that the application cycle is draining and all you want is a break (believe me, I do), but getting licensed will never be easier than when you are fresh out of school. You will never have a summer again that is completely absent of obligations other than medical school matriculation tasks. I recommend you prepare for your boards throughout your second semester of PY4 and take them as soon as possible after graduation. By doing so, you will have ample time to relax before you start medical school. You also will not have time during medical school to prepare for your NAPLEX or your state specific MPJE.

WORKING DURING MEDICAL SCHOOL:

As you adjust to medical school you may also find yourself available to work as a pharmacist. I personally recommend you do, but your school responsibilities come first. Every online resource you will find will most likely advocate for the exact opposite. "Avoid working, focus on your studies, and do research instead." While those words of advice hold true, you will find yourself having more than enough time to work a shift here and there throughout the semester. Working during the year helps maintain your pharmacy knowledge and can be a great contribution to your medical school resume. Hardly any students will work throughout medical school, so doing so will help set you apart when applying to residencies. If there are some students working, none of them will be licensed medical professionals treating real patients, which will make your application quite unique. Also, the additional pharmacy income can help resolve financial pressure during the expensive medical school semester.

If you decide that you would like to work, consider doing so AFTER your first semester is complete. Like everything, you will want an adjustment period to get used to new medical school challenges. Once you have demonstrated that you can handle the workload (which I am confident you can), look for a casual pharmacist position. If you are still wary about doing so, I recommend you wait until the summer between your M1 and M2 year. This will be a great time to get adjusted to being a practicing pharmacist with minimal medical school obligations. As you progress through the year you will realize that you can take on more and more responsibilities and you will be amazed how much you can do.

PHARMACY SCHOOL V.S. MEDICAL SCHOOL:

As you gear up for the big dance, or should I say medical school, you are probably wondering how it compares to your previous schooling. The age-old question, and a rather controversial point of discussion, is this: **"Is medical school harder than pharmacy school?"** In all honesty I beleive they are very similar and equally challenging. I can only say this about the first year of medical school. I have several more years to go before I can unrefutably claim that they are equal.

Medical school does have some different challenges, but the sheer volume of coursework and newfound responsibility is very similar to my pharmacy school experience. Most medical students will claim that medical school is the hardest education they have ever had, and that success requires substantially more work than they ever imagined. While that may be true, they probably didn't graduate with a pharmacy doctorate. You will find yourself unsurprisingly well prepared for the vigor and volume presented to you.

The only frustrating part of first year is the severe lack of clinical material you are expected to learn. Your first semester may be the most challenging solely because of the content covered. The material consists of higher-level undergraduate biology principles and anatomy instead of focusing on clinical medicine. These courses include gross anatomy, fundamentals of medicine and general chemistry-based classes. These courses hardly use your pharmacy background, which can be discouraging yet entirely manageable.

The major distinction between medical school and pharmacy school is curriculum set-up and duration of the semester. Medical schools will be highly variable when it comes to curriculum set-up but in general most classes are presented in block-style. You will focus on one major unit at a time while pharmacy tends to focus on multiple units but in less detail. The detail shifts from pharmacology, dosing, and kinetics to pathology, diagnostic criteria, and medical management. The medical school semester also tends to last slightly longer than the pharmacy curriculum, which is approximately 6 weeks shorter. An extra 6 weeks may not seem significant but after 5 months of grueling schoolwork every extra day takes its toll!

In the end, pharmacy school was more than enough to prepare me personally for the rigors of getting a medical school education. At no point during my first academic year did I feel overburdened or stressed beyond control. Pharmacy school and difficult APPE rotations make the work of medical school seem all too familiar. I am confident that you will do great, and ultimately become fantastic physicians.

PREPARING FOR THE WORST:

While this book is primarily focused on getting you into medical school there will always be a few applicants who might not get accepted. **Fear not, at the end of the day, you are still a pharmacist!** While your personal ego may have taken a hit, you will still have the opportunity for an excellent career with a six-figure salary – A far better position than some of the unsuccessful biology major applicants. Keep in mind that this isn't the end of the road. You can always re-apply! If you find yourself in this position, you should contact the medical schools you received rejections from and ask for recommendations or criticism. Some programs are excited to provide feedback and any insight can be very constructive.

Before you reapply, you need to be realistic about your application health. If you received several interview invites during your recent application cycle it's safe to say that you were almost successful. A few minor adjustments and a stronger interview and you will land an acceptance. Alternatively, if you received no interviews and plenty of early rejections in the cycle, there were major shortcomings concerning your application. Take some time and reassess what went wrong. Was it your mediocre MCAT score, your limited clinical experiences, the timing of your application, or poorly written secondaries? You will have to ask yourself these questions and be honest. If you end up reapplying, you will need to rewrite your personal statement. Almost every medical school will expect a new personal statement! I hope that none of you will have to read this particular section. **I wrote a book on how NOT to end up here.**

ADDITIONAL RESOURCES:

MD-PHD PROGRAM:

I want to introduce this unique pathway some students take to obtain a dual-doctorate and in your case, a triple doctorate. When applying through AMCAS you will be prompted with the option to choose several dual-degree education pathways. The vast majority of you will have selected the traditional M.D. path alone. While browsing the other options you will have noticed the MD-PhD pathway. This is an extremely competitive position to apply for in which most medical schools only offer 1-4 seats per class.

The program structure is as follows. You will matriculate into medical school and complete your first 2 years of education alongside your fellow class M.D. students. After completing your boards at the end of your MS2 year, you will NOT continue to rotations. Instead, you will enter the Ph.D. Portion of the program where you will spend 3-4 years working towards your doctorate in a particular research field. At the completion of your Ph.D., you will resume your medical school education as an MS3 on rotations. You will finish the last 2 years of medical school to obtain your M.D. degree.

In total this path will have doubled your time in higher education extending what was a 4 year education into an 8 year education. You may be wondering why would anyone ever do this? The major upside is that you will attend medical school for free. Take a look at the various pros and cons listed below. I don't anticipate this will be a popular pathway for the pharmacy graduate constituency, but it doesn't hurt to be informed.

Pros:
- Minimize debt including a fee medical school education.

- Ability to pursue a passion for research, or an opportunity to advance medical care.

- Opportunity to see medicine from both the developmental stages and clinical components.

- The dual-degree significantly helps students interested in a research career or academia.

Cons:
- Opportunity cost of lost attending salary.

- Very complicated application process including a much larger application and intense multiple day long interviews.

- Massive time investment during the Ph.D. part of the program.

- More competition for positions based on statistics, increasing your chances of not getting an acceptance. You may still be eligible for the traditional M.D. path if you designate so.

TEXAS MEDICAL & DENTAL SCHOOLS APPLICATION SERVICE (TMDSAS):

This is an online application platform specifically designed and utilized for Texas medical school applicants. For those of you whose legal residence presides outside of Texas, you will never have to look at this section again. While applicants form Texas can utilize the AMCAS portal, it is highly encouraged that they take advantage of their in-state advantage.

CARIBBEAN MEDICAL SCHOOLS:

Caribbean medical schools can seem rather enticing to a naïve applicant. They have very low acceptance standards and tend to target applicants who had an unsuccessful application cycle or individuals with very low statistics all around. These medical schools are erroneously coveted as a safe alternative for very low stat applicants to obtain an allopathic (M.D.) medical education. Graduates may hold the M.D. credentials, but they are also designated as "International Medical Graduates" (IMGs). While students who graduate from these medical schools can obtain medical licensure, the process of getting to that point is nightmarish to say the least.

What is frequently hidden by the picturesque campus backdrops and stunning weather is a far darker outcome for many students who travel beyond the U.S. border. What students need to understand is that most, if not all, of these medical schools are profit-seeking enterprises. They will charge students exorbitantly high tuition prices but offer substandard resources in comparison to U.S. schools. According to the White Coat Investor, the average cost for tuition is $67,773 per year, excluding the cost of living on a tropical island. This data only comes from the top-four Caribbean medical schools and there are approximately 56 others. The top four include Ross University ($80,298), St. George's University ($76,354), American University of the Caribbean ($64,465) and Saba University ($49,974).

These programs have a predilection for under-qualified students who may not be ready for the rigors of obtaining a medical education. These applicant victims take on massive amounts of debt and subsequently fail out of the medical school with nothing to show for it. The USMLE board pass rates are also cause for concern considering it's as low at 70% for Caribbean test takers. The attrition rates at these medical schools are horrendous and should frighten even the most desperate applicants away.

If a hardened student manages to make it to graduation, they will likely have seen hundreds of their fellow students fall behind or dropout. Upon graduation these IMG MD applicants will attempt to match to U.S. residency programs, which turns out to be another major problem. The residency match rates for Caribbean graduates are as low as 50%. That also accounts for the fact that most of these applicants will have chosen to NOT apply to competitive specialties. Let us review some important details to make sure you understand these crucial concepts.

- Students who plan on attending Caribbean medical schools are subjecting themselves to astronomically high costs of tuition.

- They receive an education that affords low medical board pass rates and students may have to repeat several years of school just to advance.

- Lastly, you have a 50/50 chance of matching into a non-competitive specialty. Based on this match statistic, there is NO GUAtakeRENTEE that you will even be able to practice medicine when you graduate. I can't think of a worse way to spend your time and money other than taking the MCAT 30+ times.

Attending a Caribbean medical school should be reserved as a last resort for most traditional applicants. Since you are a pharmacy student and soon to be licensed pharmacist, if you are considering a Caribbean education, I would advise you to pack-up the medical school dream. I don't mean to be discouraging, but if you are unable to obtain acceptance to either a U.S. M.D. or D.O. medical school after several application attempts, it may be time to move on! You already have a phenomenal career ahead of you and taking this route can ruin you financially, especially with such a low chance of future payout. To be fair, if there is any applicant that is qualified to make it through the rigors of Caribbean medical school, it is certainly a pharmacy graduate. I just want you to know that these programs are not as altruistic as they appear. Steer clear if you know what is good for you!

MUST READ SUPPLEMENTAL CONTENT:

As a final farewell, I recommend that you read each of these resources. The greatest minds read every day and so should you. Reading books can be a great conversation starter and major point of discussion on interviews.

1. **PharmD to MD: How to Make the Switch in Pharmacy School – Tess Calcagno, PharmD**
   https://www.studentdoctor.net/2019/05/24/pharmd-to-md/

2. **The White Coat Investor – James Dahle, MD**
   https://www.amazon.com/White-Coat-Investor-Personal-Investing/dp/0991433106

3. **Seven Figure Pharmacist – Tim Church, PharmD; Tim Ulbrich, PharmD**
   https://www.sevenfigurepharmacist.com/

4. **When Breath Becomes Air – Paul Kalanathi, MD**
   https://www.amazon.com/When-Breath-Becomes-Paul-Kalanithi/dp/081298840X

5. **The Emperor of All Maladies – Siddhartha Mukherjee, MD**
   http://siddharthamukherjee.com/the-emperor-of-all-maladies/

6. **Being Mortal: Medicine and What Matters in the End – Atul Gawande, MD**
   http://atulgawande.com/book/being-mortal/

PHARM.D. TO M.D.

CLOSING REMARKS:

I hope that this book has served you well in your endeavors and has effectively guided you through this complicated application cycle. If I can help just one student make the transition, then this book will have been a success.

I would like to take this opportunity to specially thank my personal mentors, Dr. Brandon Smith, PharmD, MD; Dr. Thomas Wright Ph.D; and Dr. Tess Calcagno, PharmD. Their contributions and insight have made this all possible. For that I am eternally grateful!

I would like to especially thank my loving family and friends who encouraged me to stay on the path, and to never falter in my convictions. I would like to thank my fellow pharmacy friends, particularly Dr. Bryce Grohol, PharmD, for suffering with me during the medical school application process. A final thanks to my loving girlfriend Julia whose patience and support throughout the production of this book has given me the necessary drive to finish this work.

Thank you for reading this book! If you felt that this resource provided you value, I kindly ask that you pass it on to others. If you have a positive story to share because of reading this book, I would love to know about it! Please feel free to email me at **PharmDtoMD2020@gmail.com** or leave a review on Amazon.

Your feedback is very important and will be used to make future editions of this book even better! If you have any suggestions, errors to report, or general feedback, please send me a message.

PHARM.D. TO M.D.

ABOUT THE AUTHOR:

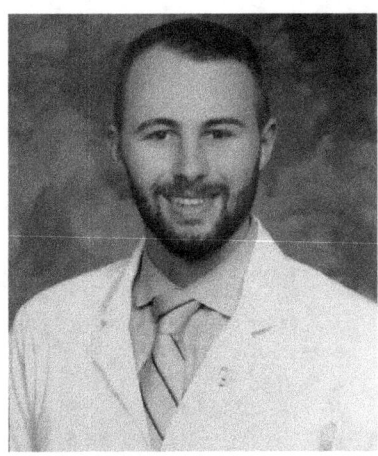

Nathan M. Gartland, PharmD

Dr. Nathan Gartland is a licensed and practicing pharmacist in New York State, as well as a second-year allopathic medical student.

After successfully completing the medical school application cycle, Nathan is working to empower other pharmacy students and graduates alike to extend their education beyond the traditional limit. He is currently interested in pursuing a career in emergency medicine or neurological surgery.

Nathan lives in Western New York with his girlfriend, Julia, and their new labrador puppy, Winston.

PHARM.D. TO M.D.

CHAPTER REFERENCES:

PART ONE: THE MEDICAL SCHOOL BLUEPRINT

1. Jessica Freedman, "Medical School Average GPA & MCAT, Admissions Statistics and Acceptance Rates (2021)." MedEdits, accessed July 7, 2021, https://mededits.com/medical-school-admissions/statistics/.

2. "GPA Calculator," Medical School Headquarters, accessed July 7, 2021, GPA Calculator (medicalschoolhq.net)

3. "LIZZYM SCORE CALCULATOR – WHAT ARE MY CHANCES FOR MEDICAL SCHOOL?" STUDENT DOCTOR NETWORK (SDN), ACCESSED JULY 7, 2021, https://www.studentdoctor.net/schools/lizzym-score

4. "Medical School Applications Cost Estimator," Medical School Headquarters, accessed July 22, 2021, https://medicalschoolhq.net/medical-school-applications-cost-estimator/

5. "Healthcare School Scholarships." goarmy.com, accessed July 7, 2021, https://www.goarmy.com/amedd/education/hpsp.html.

6. Stortz SK, Foglia LM, Thagard AS, Staat B, Lutgendorf MA. "Comparing Compensation of U.S. Military Physicians and Civilian Physicians in Residency Training and Beyond." Cureus. 2021;13(1):e12931. Published 2021 Jan 27. doi:10.7759/cureus.12931

7. "Pharmacists: Occupational Outlook Handbook." U.S. Bureau of Labor Statistics, accessed July 7, 2021, https://www.bls.gov/ooh/healthcare/mobile/pharmacists.htm.

8. "What family physicians are earning." FPM Journal, American Association of Family Physicians, accessed July 7, 2021, https://www.aafp.org/journals/fpm/blogs/inpractice/entry/physician_income.html

9. Melanie Hanson, "Average Medical School Debt." EducationData, accessed July 7, 2021, https://educationdata.org/average-medical-school-debt.

10. "Orthopedic Surgeon Salary in the United States," Salary.com, accessed July 7, 2021, https://www.salary.com/research/salary/alternate/orthopedic-surgeon-salary.

11. "Tomorrow's Doctors, Tomorrow's Cures," AAMC, accessed July 7, 2021, https://www.aamc.org/

PART TWO: THE SCHEDULE

12. "How Long Are MCAT® Scores Valid?" AAMC, accessed July 8, 2021, https://students-residents.aamc.org/mcat-scores/how-long-are-mcat-scores-valid

13. "Medical School Requirements in 2021: The Definitive Guide, Learn what medical school prerequisites to take and what extracurricular activities to pursue to meet your pre med requirements and maximize your admission chances, Shemmassian Academic Consulting, accessed July 8, 2021, https://www.shemmassianconsulting.com/blog/medical-school-requirements#medical-school-course-requirements

14. "Undergraduate Tuition Rates," Duquesne University, accessed July 8, 2021, https://duq.edu/admissions-and-aid/tuition/undergraduate-tuition-rates

15. "Guidelines for Writing a Letter of Evaluation for a Medical School Applicant (PDF)," AAMC, accessed July 8, 2021, https://www.aamc.org/system/files?file=2019-09/lettersguidelinesbrochure.pdf

16. "Early Decision Program," AAMC, accessed July 8, 2021, Early Decision Program | AAMC

17. "Should You Apply Early Decision to Medical School?" The Princeton Review, accessed July 8, 2021, Should You Apply Early Decision to Medical School? | The Princeton Review

18. "How to Get Into the Wake Forest School of Medicine: Requirements and Strategies," Shemmassian Academic Counseling, accessed July 8, 2021, https://www.shemmassianconsulting.com/blog/wake-forest-school-of-medicine#:~:text=Wake%20Forest%20Medical%20School%20sets,to%20reach%20the%20admissions%20committee.

PART THREE: THE MCAT

19. "Summary of MCAT Total and Section Scores," AAMC, accessed July 8, 2021, https://students-residents.aamc.org/media/8356/download

20. "Khan Academy Test Prep MCAT," Khan Academy, accessed July 17, 2021, https://www.khanacademy.org/test-prep/mcat

21. "MCAT – Medical School Admission Test," r/MCAT, Reddit, accessed July 17, 2021, https://www.reddit.com/r/Mcat/wiki/index

22. "Free MCAT Exam & Other Resources." Blueprint, accessed July 17, 2021, https://blueprintprep.com/mcat/free-resources/free-mcat-practice-bundle

23. "Jack Westin CARS Passages," Jack Westin Prep, accessed July 18, 2021, https://jackwestin.com/mcat-question-of-the-day

24. "MCAT Test Preparation Courses and Packages." The Princeton Review, accessed July 18, 2021, https://www.princetonreview.com/medical/mcat-test-prep?ceid=newhp-nav

25. "MCAT Preparation." UWorld, accessed July 18, 2021, https://www.uworld.com/collegeprep/mcat/mcat.aspx

26. Kevin Wang, "Thinking About Voiding Your MCAT? Here's What You Should Know." Med School Tutors, accessed July 21, 2021, https://www.medschooltutors.com/blog/thinking-about-voiding-your-mcat-heres-what-you-should

PART FOUR: THE PRIMARY APPLICATION

27. "Medical School Letters of Recommendation," The Princeton Review, accessed July 8, 2021, https://www.princetonreview.com/med-school-advice/med-school-recommendations

28. Rob Humbracht, "Every Question You Have About Letters of Recommendation for Medical School," The Savvy Pre-Med, accessed July 8, 2021, https://www.savvypremed.com/blog/every-question-you-have-about-letters-of-recommendation-for-medical-school-1

29. "2021 AMCAS Applicant Guide (PDF)," AAMC, accessed July 8, 2021, https://students-residents.aamc.org/media/5186/download

30. William Burnett. "Legal Matters: Institutional Action Basics." The Student Doctor Network, accessed July 21, 2021, https://www.studentdoctor.net/2020/02/13/legal-matters-institutional-action-basics/

31. "AMCAS® Application Course Classification Guide (PDF)," AAMC, accessed July 21, 2021, https://students-residents.aamc.org/media/7861/download

32. "2021 AMCAS Work and Activities Ultimate Guide (Examples Included)," Shemassian Academic Consulting, accessed July 21, 2021, https://www.shemmassianconsulting.com/blog/amcas-work-and-activities#amcas-work-and-activities-categories=

33. "AMCAS Most Meaningful Experience: What You Need To Know For 2021." Cracking Med School Admissions, accessed July 21, 2021, https://crackingmedadmissions.com/amcas-most-meaningful-experience/

34. "Dossier." Interfolio, accessed July 22, 2021, https://www.interfolio.com/products/dossier/?gclid=Cj0KCQjwx7zzBRCcARIsABPRscO2qZHhqeEqaI0bbLWfUCz363Q2EbqBVJuMhIl8h3mw51w4Vtc9Gn4aAvZZEALw_wcB#signup

35. Lauren Jarvis, "Feature Spotlight: Gaaranteed quality check on all letters." Interfolio, accessed July 22, 2021, https://www.interfolio.com/resources/blog/quality-check-on-letters/

36. "How to: Use Dossier Deliver for a medical or dental school application." Interfolio, accessed July 22, 2021, https://support.interfolio.com/m/62586/l/646844-how-to-use-dossier-deliver-for-a-medical-or-dental-school-application

37. "Medical School Admission Requirements™ for Applicants." AAMC, accessed July 22, 2021, https://students-residents.aamc.org/medical-school-admission-requirements/medical-school-admission-requirements-applicants

38. "The Cost of Applying to Medical School." AAMC, accessed July 22, 2021, https://students-residents.aamc.org/financial-aid-resources/cost-applying-medical-school

39. "How Many Medical Schools Should I Apply To? Which Ones?" Shemmassian Academic Consulting, accessed July 22, 2021, https://www.shemmassianconsulting.com/blog/how-many-medical-schools-should-i-apply-to#part-3-how-many-medical-schools-should-i-apply-to=

40. Kathleen Franco, "7 Tips for Nailing Medical School Letters of Recommendation." U.S. News, accessed July 8, 2021, https://www.usnews.com/education/blogs/medical-school-admissions-doctor/2015/04/14/7-tips-for-nailing-medical-school-letters-of-recommendation

41. "Medical School Acceptance Rates: In-State vs. Out-of-State" Accepted, accessed July 8, 2021, https://www.accepted.com/medical/in-state-out-of-state-admissions

42. "Building a List of Schools," Pre-Med Hub – University of Michigan, accessed July 8, 2021, https://premedhubumich.com/1977-2/

43. "2021 Medical School Personal Statement Ultimate Guide (Examples Included)." Shemmassian Academic Consulting, accessed July 22, 2021, https://www.shemmassianconsulting.com/blog/medical-school-personal-statement-analysis#part-2-a-step-by-step-approach-to-writing-an-amazing-medical-school-personal-statement=

44. Gyubari. "Writing Your Personal Statement: A How-To." Reddit, accessed July 22, 2021, https://www.reddit.com/r/premed/comments/fh3s2y/writing_your_personal_statement_a_howto/

45. Josh Moody, "10 Most Expensive Private Medical Schools." U.S. News, accessed July 8, 2021, https://www.usnews.com/education/best-graduate-schools/the-short-list-grad-school/articles/most-expensive-private-medical-schools

46. Emma Kerr, "10 Public Med Schools With Low Out-of-State Costs." U.S. News, accessed July 8, 2021, https://www.usnews.com/education/best-graduate-schools/the-short-list-grad-school/articles/most-affordable-medical-schools-for-out-of-state-students

PART FIVE: SECONDARY APPLICATIONS

47. Ryan Kelly, "The Five Most Common Medical School Secondary Essay Prompts for 2018." The Savvy Pre-Med, accessed July 8, 2021, https://www.savvypremed.com/blog/the-five-most-common-medical-school-secondary-essay-prompts-for-2018

48. Edward Chang, "Secondary Application Practical Advice." Prospective Doctor, accessed July 8, 2021, https://www.prospectivedoctor.com/secondary-application-practical-advice/

49. "Medical School Secondary Essay Prompts Database." Prospective Doctor, accessed July 22, 2021, https://www.prospectivedoctor.com/medical-school-secondary-essay-prompts-database/

50. "Medical School Secondary Essays: The Complete Guide (Examples Included)." Shemmassian Academic Consulting, accessed July 8, 2021, https://www.shemmassianconsulting.com/blog/medical-school-secondary-essays#part-2-the-medical-school-diversity-essay

51. Ryan Kelly, "Do's and Don'ts for Writing About Coronavirus in Your Personal Statement." The Savvy Pre-Med, accessed July 8, 2021, https://www.savvypremed.com/blog/dos-and-donts-for-writing-about-coronavirus-in-your-personal-statement

PART SIX: THE CAPSER EXAM

52. "Altus Suite (Casper, Snapshot, & Duet) School List for the 2021-2022 Cycle." Reddit, accessed July 22, 2021, https://www.reddit.com/r/premed/wiki/casper/casperschools

53. "How to Prepare for the Casper Test to Get Into Medical School." Shemmassian Academic Consulting, accessed July 8, 2021, https://www.shemmassianconsulting.com/blog/casper-test#part-1-introduction

54. "CASPer, Duet, and Snapshot: The Facts (2021-2022)." MedEdits Medical Admissions, accessed July 22, 2021, https://mededits.com/medical-school-application/casper-test-prep-2019-2020/#List_of_Medical_Schools_that_Require_CASPer,_Snapshot_and_Duet_ (updated_as_of_July,_2021)

55. "Altus Suite: Casper, Snapshot, and Duet." r/premed, Reddit, accessed July 8, 2021, https://www.reddit.com/r/premed/wiki/casper#wiki_what_is_altus_suite.3F

56. "What is Altus Suite?" Altus Suite, accessed July 8, 2021, https://takealtus.com/

57. "How the CASPer Test is Scored." BeMo Academic Consulting, accessed July 8, 2021, https://bemoacademicconsulting.com/blog/how-is-casper-test-scored

58. "Key CASPer Test Question Categories and CASPer Test Question Types." BeMo Academic Consulting, accessed July 22, 2021, https://bemoacademicconsulting.com/blog/casper-test-question-categories-and-types

59. "Sample CASPer® Questions." Astroff, accessed July 22, 2021, https://www.caspertest.com/casper-sample-questions/

60. "Hot to maximize your chances of success on Casper." Altus Suite, accessed July 8, 2021, https://takealtus.com/2020/07/how-to-maximize-your-chances-of-success-on-casper/

61. "Duet by Altus: Your Comprehensive 2021 Prep Guide." BeMo Academic Consulting, accessed July 8, 2021, https://bemoacademicconsulting.com/blog/duet

62. "AAMC Situational Judgment Test (SJT)." Reddit, accessed July 22, 2021, https://www.reddit.com/r/premed/wiki/sjt/

63. "AAMC SJT Participating Medical Schools." AAMC, accessed July 22, 2021, https://students-residents.aamc.org/aamc-situational-judgment-test/participating-medical-schools

PART SEVEN: OSTEOPATHIC SCHOOLS OF MEDICINE

64. "Is M.D. Better Than D.O.." Prospective Doctor, accessed July 8, 2021, https://www.prospectivedoctor.com/is-md-better-than-do/

65. "The Best Osteopathic Medical Schools: DO School Rankings List." Shemmassian Academic Consulting, accessed July 8, 2021, https://www.shemmassianconsulting.com/blog/best-do-schools

66. "U.S. Colleges of Osteopathic Medicine." AACOM® Choose DO, A New Generation of Doctors, accessed July 8, 2021, https://choosedo.org/us-colleges-of-osteopathic-medicine/#:~:text=There%20are%20currently%2037%20accredited,of%20all%20U.S.%20medical%20students.

67. "2021 AACOMAS Application Guide For DO Schools," Med School Insiders, accessed July 8, 2021, https://medschoolinsiders.com/pre-med/aacomas-application-guide/

68. "College Application Deadlines for 2021 Entering Class." AACOM® Choose DO, A New Generation of Doctors, accessed July 22, 2021, https://choosedo.org/college-application-deadlines/

69. Edward Chang, "Should I Apply to DO schools?" Prospective Doctor, accessed July 8, 2021, https://www.prospectivedoctor.com/should-i-apply-to-do-schools/

70. Kasey Isaacs, "What are the differences between an MD and a DO?" Atlantis, accessed July 8, 2021, https://joinatlantis.com/blog/md-vs-do-which-is-right-for-you/

71. "MD vs DO: The Biggest Differences (And Which is Better)." Shemmassian Academic Consulting, accessed July 8, 2021, https://www.shemmassianconsulting.com/blog/md-vs-do-admissions-what-are-the-differences

72. "Main Residency Math Data and Reports," The Match: National Residency Matching Program, accessed July 8, 2021, https://www.nrmp.org/main-residency-match-data/

PART EIGHT: THE INTERVIEW

73. "How to Ace Medical School Interviews (Questions Included)." Shemmassian Academic Consulting, accessed July 8, 2021, https://www.shemmassianconsulting.com/blog/medical-school-interviews#part-1-introduction-medical-school-interviews

74. "Interview Feedback," The Student Doctor Network (SDN), accessed July 8, 2021, https://www.studentdoctor.net/schools/schools/12/allopathic-medical-school-interview-feedback/1

75. "Types of Medical School Interviews," Ingenious Prep, accessed July 8, 2021, https://ingeniusprep.com/blog/types-of-medical-school-interviews/

76. "5 Common Med School Interview Questions and How to Answer Them." Medical School Headquarters, accessed July 8, 2021, https://medicalschoolhq.net/pmy-233-5-common-med-school-interview-questions-and-how-to-answer-them/

77. Giulia Bankov, "How to prepare for medical school interview: The Group Task." The Medical School Application Guide (MSAG), accessed July 8, 2021, https://themsag.com/blogs/medical-school-interviews/how-to-prepare-for-medical-school-interview-the-group-task

78. "What it's like to Participate in Multiple Mini Interviews (MMIs)." AAMC, accessed July 8, 2021, https://students-residents.aamc.org/applying-medical-school/what-it-s-participate-multiple-mini-interviews-mmis

79. "MMI Interview: The Ultimate Guide (150 Sample Questions Included)." Shemmassian Academic Consulting, accessed July 22, 2021, https://www.shemmassianconsulting.com/blog/mmi-interview#mmi-interview-prep=

PART NINE: THE PRE/POST-INTERVIEW LIMBO

80. "Every Question You Have About Medical School Waitlists." The Savvy Pre-Med, accessed July 8, 2021, https://www.savvypremed.com/blog/every-question-you-have-about-medical-school-waitlists

81. "How to Write an Effective Letter of Intent for Medical School." The Savvy Pre-Med, accessed July 8, 2021, https://www.savvypremed.com/blog/how-to-write-an-effective-letter-of-intent-for-medical-school

PART TEN: HOLDING A MEDICAL SCHOOL ACCEPTANCE

82. "What to Do After Getting Accepted Into Medical School." Med School Coach, accessed July 8, 2021, https://www.medschoolcoach.com/what-to-do-after-getting-accepted-into-medical-school/

83. "AMCAS® Choose Your Medical School Tool." AAMC, accessed July 8, 2021, https://students-residents.aamc.org/prehealth-advisors/amcas-choose-your-medical-school-tool

84. "Reapplying to Medical School: Every Major Question Answered." Shemmassian Academic Consulting, accessed July 8, 2021, https://www.shemmassianconsulting.com/blog/reapplying-to-medical-school

ADDITIONAL RESOURCES

85. James Dahle, "How To Choose A Medical Or Dental School." The White Coat Investor's Guide for Students. WCI Intellectual Property, LLC. 2021. Accessed July 22, 2021

86. "Caribbean Medical Schools: What You Need to Know." Medical School Headquarters, accessed July 22, 2021, https://medicalschoolhq.net/caribbean-medical-schools-what-you-need-to-know/

87. Tess Calcagno, "PharmD to MD: How to Make the Switch in Pharmacy School." The Student Doctor Network, accessed July 22, 2021, https://www.studentdoctor.net/2019/05/24/pharmd-to-md/

www.ingramcontent.com/pod-product-compliance
Lightning Source LLC
Chambersburg PA
CBHW060828220526
45466CB00003B/1015